THE COMPLETE ALLERGY-FREE COMFORT FOODS COOKBOOK

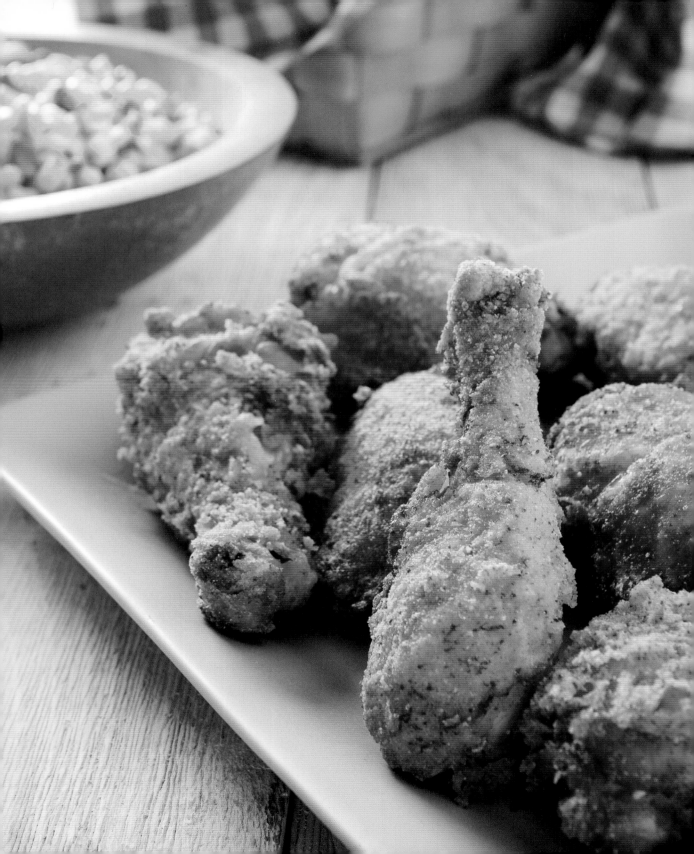

THE **COMPLETE ALLERGY-FREE COMFORT FOODS COOKBOOK**

EVERY RECIPE IS FREE OF GLUTEN, DAIRY, SOY, NUTS, AND EGGS

ELIZABETH GORDON

PHOTOGRAPHY BY SUSAN BYRNES

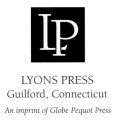

LYONS PRESS
Guilford, Connecticut
An imprint of Globe Pequot Press

{ For Margot, Colombe, and Jesse, who make my life sweet every day, and for sweet Blossom, who was so excited to become the next great chef }

To buy books in quantity for corporate use or incentives, call **(800) 962-0973** or e-mail **premiums@GlobePequot.com.**

Lyons Press is an imprint of Globe Pequot Press.

Photography by Susan Byrnes

Text design: Sheryl Kober

Layout artist: Kevin Fall

Project editor: Gregory Hyman/Kristen Mellitt

ISBN 978-0-7627-8813-2

Printed in the United States of America

10 9 8 7 6 5 4 3 2 1

Library of Congress Cataloging-in-Publication Data is available on file.

Contents

Introduction

When I was diagnosed with food allergies in 2004, my oldest daughter was a baby who hadn't even started solid foods. Of course the news that I wouldn't be able to eat eggs, wheat, or string beans again was shocking (well, maybe not the string beans part), and I thought that I would never be able to eat anything tasty again. I adapted. I started baking for my allergies, and I created desserts that my insatiable sweet tooth loved.

However, as my children get older, cooking plays a more central role in our lives. I find cooking for the family far more challenging than baking for us. At first I cooked different dinners for all of us, but the dazzle of working as a short-order line chef quickly wore off. Growing up, my family ate dinner together every single night, and it was important to me to continue this tradition. We always ate family-style and talked about our day, and I not only wanted to do the same with my own family, but I also worried about the psychological repercussions of having two daughters who watched their mother eat something different from their meal every night. I wanted us not only to commune as a family but also to be able to partake in the same dinner. I wanted our entire family to be able to experience all of the regional dishes that I grew up with living in Ohio, Tennessee, and, later, Germany, France, and New York.

Relishing a challenge, I set out to make allergy-friendly versions of the comfort foods of my youth. However, when I started thinking about recipes and asking other people about their experiences with cooking for food allergies, many complained that eating with food allergies gets pricey, so I have tried to create recipes that are safe and delicious but that won't break the bank. I have discovered that the allergy-friendly prepared foods are what get expensive, but that if I cook my own meals instead of reaching for prepared crackers or frozen gluten-free waffles, I can actually keep our grocery bill pretty close to what it was before I was diagnosed with food allergies.

I hope that by sharing these recipes with you, you will find gluten-, dairy-, soy-, nut-, and egg-free eating less expensive than you expected. A couple of the ingredients, like xanthan gum and some of the flours, are more expensive than traditional all-purpose flour, but when stored properly, they last for a very long time, which makes them economical in the long run. In terms of the main courses in the book, I use less expensive cuts of meat like pork shoulder, chuck roast, and ground beef to save you money, and the vegetarian selections are almost always less expensive than a dinner made with meat. Rice and potatoes are never expensive, and yet both are high in fiber and healthier than processed wheat pasta. There are always little ways to save, too, like freezing leftover coconut milk kefir in single-serve containers rather than letting the remainder go bad in the refrigerator, or making your own chicken stock instead of buying it off the shelf at the supermarket. Just remember that some ingredients may be slightly more expensive, but you are paying for safety, peace of mind, and, in some cases, additional nutrition.

As you leaf through the pages of this book, you will see enticing photos of delicious dishes that are, for the most part, quick and healthy. However, a couple of gasp-worthy methods and terms may jump out at you: I use lard and coconut milk in this book. I also fry a few things, though I do not fry them in lard but use canola oil instead. I know that using lard is antithetical to everything nutritionists nationwide tell us to eat to lose weight. However, they are not chefs, and they, therefore, do not appreciate the fact that leaf lard makes the flakiest piecrusts and keeps a gluten-, dairy-, soy-, nut-, and egg-free pastry and some kinds of cookies from being tough. I also want to stress that cookies and pies and fried chicken are treats. My family loves to pack up a box of fried chicken for a summer beach picnic, and I love to serve my Mint Thin Wafers now and then, but I don't serve these items every day of the week. Sweet treats punctuate the end of a meal; they are not the main event.

As for the coconut, after speaking with several well-known allergists, severely nut-allergic friends, and parents of severely nut-allergic children, I decided to include it. Though the Food and Drug Administration (FDA) classifies coconut as a tree nut, most of the medical community seems to agree that it is part of the palm family and that most, but not all, nut-allergy sufferers can safely consume it. If this is not the case for your family, I have included a substitution guide, and you should be able to find something that works for you. As always, I encourage you to check with your doctor before using any new ingredient, and as I like to say: When in doubt, leave it out.

I hope that your family enjoys these recipes as much as mine. There is nothing more satisfying to me as a busy mom than coming home, whipping up something quick, and not hearing a single complaint from the table. I wanted to share these recipes with you so that your mealtimes can go from stressful to stress-free and to show you that just because you or your loved one may have multiple food allergies, you do not have to sacrifice taste, variety, or fun with food.

What the Heck?: An Allergy-Free Dictionary of Ingredients

Baking and cooking for food allergies is really easy, but it does require an entirely new list of ingredients that may leave you scratching your head. Once you familiarize yourself with the names of the ingredients and their purposes, combining them to make your favorite dishes and desserts is simple. Despite the fact that you may never have used any of these ingredients before, we are lucky that, today, most of these ingredients are readily available in supermarkets nationwide. If you still have trouble finding the following ingredients, never fear: The Internet is just a click away and so, therefore, are any missing ingredients! Check the Where to Shop section at the back of this book to find places to buy all the ingredients you will need to get started.

Bouquet Garni—A bouquet garni is simply a bunch of fresh herbs tied together with a bit of the dark part of a leek. Bouquet garni is often used to infuse flavors into soups and stocks and is fished out and discarded before serving.

Chinese or Superfine Rice Flour—When I first started cooking and baking my way around my egg and wheat allergies, I steered clear of rice flour unless I was making something that needed to be grainy. Most rice flours are ground fine, but not fine enough to go unnoticed in a recipe. But then, a couple of years ago, a friend of mine introduced me to Chinese rice flour. She gets it in Chinatown or from her Korean greengrocer, and it is so much cheaper than any other gluten-free flours that I am familiar with! However, not all of us live near Chinatown or a Korean greengrocer, so also look for "superfine" rice flour. The best part of Chinese or superfine rice flour is that it not only has a neutral flavor but also a smooth texture that does not leave baked goods tasting gritty. When I refer to superfine or Chinese rice flour, I am always referring to the white variety. Superfine brown rice flour weighs more and will change the outcome of your recipe. See the Where to Shop section for brand names and where to purchase them.

Cider Vinegar—I use cider vinegar in my baking recipes to activate the baking soda and as a tenderizer in recipes like fried chicken. Even in the recipes that call for coconut milk kefir, I usually add a tablespoon of cider vinegar, even though it's not entirely necessary, to add extra volume to the cake or quick bread. Don't worry: You will not be able to taste the vinegar in the finished product, or even in the batter.

Coconut Milk—In this book I use two different kinds of coconut milk: canned and the kind you find in the dairy aisle. Coconut milk is nondairy, and I use the canned variety in things like curry, where it is desirable to taste the coconut flavor, or in chocolate frosting, where the chocolate masks the flavor. I use the other kind of coconut milk, the kind you find in the dairy section that comes in "milk" cartons, when I want to achieve creaminess but do not want to taste the coconut flavor. So Delicious brand coconut milk is a terrific stand in for milk or cream, and I love that it is lower in fat and calories and devoid of the flavor found in the canned variety.

Coconut Milk Kefir—In my first book, *Allergy-Free Desserts: Gluten-Free, Dairy-Free, Egg-Free, Soy-Free and Nut-Free Delights*, I made "buttermilk" from cider vinegar and rice milk, and you can continue to do so in these recipes if that feels like a better fit for you. However, I recently discovered coconut milk kefir in the dairy aisle at my local supermarket. It is an excellent substitute for traditional buttermilk in baking recipes, and it requires no additional mixing.

Dairy- and Soy-Free Margarine—What do you do when you can't eat butter? Well, if you are baking, then you use organic palm fruit oil shortening. However, if you want to make cinnamon toast, for example, then I recommend using Earth Balance dairy- and soy-free margarine. It has the best taste of the brands that I have had, and it is easy to find in most Whole Foods and local supermarkets nationwide.

Dark Chocolate—There are a couple of recipes in which I recommend using squares of very dark chocolate. I recommend chocolates that are 70 percent cocoa or higher, because they are usually free of both dairy and soy; however, this is not always the case, so be sure to carefully read ingredients labels before you buy. Also, though most companies have stringent protocol in place with regard to washing their equipment before running a dairy- and soy-free line, there is still a very small risk of cross-contamination. If you have very severe allergies and the threat of cross-contamination is too risky, then I recommend using the Enjoy Life dairy- and soy-free chocolate chips in place of the squares of dark chocolate.

Flaxseed Meal—Flaxseed meal is simply ground flaxseeds, but in allergy-free baking it makes an excellent egg substitute. I especially love to use flaxseed meal in cookies, because its naturally nutty flavor enhances the flavor of most recipes. As an added bonus, flaxseeds are high in omega-3 fatty acids, which are great for heart health. One tablespoon of flaxseed meal mixed with three tablespoons of water stands in for one egg in most baked recipes.

French Lentils—Smaller than their red counterparts, French lentils are a green variety of lentil. I like to use them when making lentil stews, because they tend to be firmer and don't get mushy during cooking.

Gluten-, Dairy-, Soy-, Nut-, and Egg-Free Chocolate Chips—Cocoa powder is naturally dairy- and soy-free, but the chocolate chips we're accustomed to baking with are not. Most chocolate in this country is emulsified, or bound, with cocoa butter (which is dairy-free) and soy lecithin. Some people with soy allergies can still tolerate soy lecithin, but not everyone can, so I prefer to work with soy-free chocolate. You can buy dairy- and soy-free chocolate chips from kosher marketplaces that carry "kosher for Passover" chocolate. (Soybeans are not kosher for Passover.) However, if you are sensitive to nuts, then there is a risk of cross-contamination with kosher for Passover chocolate. If this is the case, look in your supermarket for brands that are gluten-, dairy-, soy-, nut-, and egg-free and produced in a dedicated facility, like Enjoy Life–brand chocolate chips.

Gluten-Free All-Purpose Baking Flour—In a few of my recipes, I recommend using Bob's Red Mill Gluten-Free All-Purpose Baking Flour. It has always been a favorite of mine for baking cookies, as it lends just the right texture as well as a delicious, nutty flavor to them. Fortunately, it is very easy to find at most supermarkets. However, if you cannot find it in your area, check out the company's website to have it shipped directly to you. If you feel uncomfortable with Bob's products because of possible cross-contamination issues, please see my substitutions guide for ways to work around this product. My substitutions chart provides the weights of common gluten-free flours to make substituting easier. I use Arrowhead Mills Gluten-Free All-Purpose Baking Mix in the Funnel Cakes recipe for the extra leavening and hint of cinnamon in the mix. This brand is as accessible as Bob's brand, but the two do not work interchangeably. King Arthur also makes a nice blend that is available at most supermarkets and that can be used interchangeably with the Bob's Red Mill Gluten-Free All-Purpose Baking Flour.

Gluten-Free Rice Milk—If you cannot tolerate coconut milk and decide to use rice milk in its place, make sure the rice milk you use is gluten free. Some rice milk brands contain barley, which is fine if you do not have a gluten sensitivity, but if you are gluten sensitive, make sure to pay careful attention to the ingredients list.

Leaf Lard—In most of my recipes I use organic palm fruit oil shortening. But I noticed that for a couple of them, it just wasn't providing the right texture. So, in a fit of desperation, I turned to lard, and the texture mystery was solved. Although not considered the healthiest fat, lard is bar none the best when it comes to producing a flakey piecrust or, in my case, a crisp, but not hard allergy-free sugar cookie. When using it, remember to look for nonhydrogenated varieties. Leaf lard is becoming harder to find, but it is worth the hunt. The flavor is better, and it is nonhydrogenated. Though you may find regular lard on the shelf at your local supermarket, it is usually hydrogenated and has a chemical, porky flavor. Leaf lard, or nonhydrogenated lard, has a more neutral flavor than hydrogenated lard and is usually available at most farmers' markets, or check the Where to Shop guide at the back of this book for an online outlet. If you have trouble finding it at the farmers' market and you prefer not to buy it online, ask your local butcher if he or she could source some for you. Keep in mind that I only use lard in desserts, which should always be eaten in moderation.

Lyle's Golden Syrup—I hadn't heard of Lyle's, long a British baking favorite, until I was writing my first book a few years ago. A British friend turned me on to it, and since using it, I can't get enough of it. It is a more natural stand-in for corn syrup, as it is simply sugar and water cooked down into a thick syrup. I was so pleased to see Lyle's popping up on the shelves of the supermarkets in New York City and California, but if you have trouble finding it, you can substitute light corn syrup in its place.

Maldon Salt—Maldon is a natural British sea salt that I like to use, especially in french fries and roasted potato dishes. I recommend it for its flaky, crunchy texture and the way that it adds intensity to a dish without your needing to use as much salt. It's also really pretty on the table in a salt cellar, and because it is so natural, it's the perfect complement to meals.

Masa Harina—Masa harina is a finely ground white corn flour that is used in many Latin American dishes. It is used specifically in making tortillas, pupusas, and tamales, as well as in many other Latin American recipes.

Millet Flour—Interestingly, millet is one of the oldest-known grains, dating back to Biblical times. It has been used in breads and baked goods for centuries, and I use it in my gluten-free bread to lend a delicate crumb and golden browning.

Oil Mister—I know that this is not really an ingredient, but I have found this tool to be an essential part of soy- and dairy-free cooking. Most nonstick sprays contain soy, so I like to make my very own spray with a commercial misting bottle and my own oil. Whether you choose olive oil or canola is up to you, but this handy tool will help keep your pans from sticking and help turn the tops of your potpies a gorgeous golden brown. See the Where to Shop guide about where to pick one up.

Organic Palm Fruit Oil Shortening—My mother inspired this allergy-free baking favorite. When we were growing up, everybody loved her chocolate chip cookies and always asked for the secret ingredient. What they didn't know was that it wasn't what she put in but what she left out. She never used butter in her chocolate chip cookies, but instead used shortening. So, when I decided to make dairy-free cookies, it was a snap. However, when I took my baking one step further and also turned my cookies soy free, the challenge was to find a soy-free shortening. I didn't have to look very far. I found organic palm fruit oil shortening first online, then at the health food store, and now I find it at the regular supermarket. It can be easy to miss, as most of the brands say "All-Vegetable Shortening" on the front label. Just check the list of ingredients; it usually reveals that the vegetable used in the shortening is organic palm fruit oil. Trans fat free and nonhydrogenated, palm fruit oil is soy-free (palm oil shortening is made from palm oil, not soy beans) and is a healthy alternative to traditional shortening.

Potato Starch—Like cornstarch, potato starch is an excellent thickener when used in gravies. It can also be used to replace eggs, but I use it in my baked goods because it replicates the delicate crumb you're used to eating in cakes and cookies that are not gluten-free.

Powdered Vanilla Rice Milk—This is one of my favorite discoveries, and I like to use it in frostings for added depth and flavor. The best part of powdered vanilla rice milk is the fact that it is shelf stable even after opening and, therefore, lasts for a very long time. It is more economical in this respect, and the flavor is delicious. I use it for "buttermilk" with a little cider vinegar if I'm baking for someone who is coconut intolerant or if I'm making my very favorite frosting recipe.

Sorghum Beer—Sadly, beer is glutinous, thanks to the barley and hops used to make it. Fortunately there are beers on the market that are gluten-free. I like to use sorghum beer in stews and some types of bread for added flavor and also to help with leavening.

Sorghum Flour—Sorghum is one of many kinds of gluten-free flour on the market today. Long used as a feed for animals, sorghum has experienced a newfound popularity in the United States, thanks to the number of people following a gluten-free diet. I use sorghum flour in small quantities in my baked goods because it is gluten-free, has a neutral flavor, and is denser than rice flour. With sorghum, cookies aren't too lacey and cakes still have the moist and light texture that you're used to eating in regular cakes.

Xanthan Gum—Xanthan gum is the number-one, most important ingredient in gluten-free baking. Take a close look at a piece of cake or bread and you will see tiny holes where little air bubbles formed and then burst while baking. Those little bubbles occur thanks to the gluten in regular wheat flour, and they are what create the texture of baked goods that you're used to eating. In gluten-free baking, the xanthan gum creates these little air bubbles in the absence of gluten. Without xanthan gum, your cookies will look like little puddles and your cakes will not rise, even with baking soda and baking powder. Xanthan gum is also an excellent thickener, though I prefer to use potato starch or cornstarch when thickening sauces, as xanthan will not thicken cold substances and can be gummy and slippery if not used in the right proportions.

Substitutions

The most interesting thing about what I do is neither testing new recipes nor discovering new ingredients. What I love is hearing from people who are living with food allergies and who also like to cook as much as I do. Along the way I have learned that foods that seem innocuous to one person could be deadly to another and that what is available in my neck of the woods might not be available in yours. Therefore, in this book, I wanted to include a table of substitutions, because what may work for me may not work for you. Although I am including these substitutions, the recipes in this book have only been tested using the ingredients listed in them. However, they should work just fine with these stand-ins.

Bob's Red Mill Gluten-Free All-Purpose Baking Flour—Per cup of all-purpose gluten-free baking flour, you can substitute the following mixture: $3/4$ cup superfine white rice flour plus 1 tablespoon rice flour plus $1/4$ cup plus 1 tablespoon potato starch plus 1 tablespoon plus 1 teaspoon sorghum flour. You may also substitute King Arthur Gluten-Free Multi-Purpose Flour cup for cup. The "spread," if you are making cookies, may be slightly less than with the Bob's Red Mill blend, but it should work just as well.

Chinese or Superfine White Rice Flour—Rice flour is very light in weight, so to substitute for 1 cup of rice flour, you will have to use less of other flours. You could use $3/4$ cup plus 2 tablespoons sorghum or millet flour or $3/4$ cup Bob's Red Mill All-Purpose Baking Flour or $3/4$ cup plus 2 tablespoons quinoa flour.

Cider Vinegar—If apple allergies make it impossible for you to use cider vinegar, you may substitute the same amount of lemon juice. Some leavening agents require an acid for activation, which is why the cider vinegar is in the recipe. Simply use lemon juice instead.

Coconut Milk—In most recipes, rice or soy milk can be substituted for coconut milk, though the consistency, like in a curry, will be thinner and the flavor may be lacking. In a pudding, for example, the finished product may not set up quite as well as it would with coconut milk.

Coconut Milk Kefir—If you cannot tolerate coconut or cannot find coconut milk kefir, simply use the same amount of rice milk (or nondairy milk of your choice) called for in the recipe plus 1 tablespoon cider vinegar or lemon juice.

Cornstarch—There are lots of options when substituting for cornstarch. Per 1 tablespoon of cornstarch, you can substitute 1 tablespoon of rice flour or potato flour or potato starch; 2 teaspoons arrowroot; or 1 tablespoon tapioca starch.

Flaxseed Meal—Applesauce can be substituted for flaxseed meal in most of my recipes. One-fourth cup applesauce is equal to 1 tablespoon flaxseed meal plus 3 tablespoons water.

Fryer—A fryer is not an ingredient, but I do use it in a few recipes in this book (such as onion rings), and I do consider it nearly crucial. The fryer keeps the temperature of the frying oil stable, which is more difficult to do on a stove top. If you do not have a fryer, use a large, heavy skillet filled with about 3 to 4 inches of canola oil. If you are using this method to fry, it is imperative that you use a candy thermometer, which will not melt, to constantly measure the temperature of the oil. In my recipes the oil should remain at 350°F during frying. Otherwise, if it is too hot, the food will scorch, or, if the oil is too cool, all of the coating will fall off and your onion rings will be limp.

Gluten-Free Oats—Sometimes the most sensitive tummies still can't handle certified gluten-free oats. Try substituting the same amount of quinoa flakes instead.

Lard—As I have mentioned, nothing works better at creating flakiness in a gluten-free piecrust or sugar cookie than lard. However, if you are vegetarian or cannot use lard because you are kosher, you can substitute the same amount of organic palm fruit oil shortening or soy-free margarine in a recipe. The texture will not be the same, but it will work.

Lyle's Golden Syrup—Light corn syrup can be substituted in a 1:1 ratio for Lyle's.

Organic Palm Fruit Oil Shortening—Lots of people have asked me about this one, either because they cannot find organic palm fruit oil in their area or they live outside the United States and it is not sold in their country. There are substitutes, though some contain soy. Any other kind of vegetable shortening, dairy and soy-free margarine included, may be used in place of organic palm fruit oil shortening. Crisco (in the United States), Copha (in Australia), and Trex or White Flora (in the United Kingdom) are some examples of vegetable shortenings worldwide, but as I said, they may contain soy. It seems that Pflanzenfett (in Germany) doesn't work. Vegetable suet may also be substituted for organic palm fruit oil shortening; just be sure to check the label to make certain that it doesn't contain wheat.

Pumpkin Seeds—If you cannot tolerate the pepitas in my muesli recipe, try using sunflower seeds instead.

Sorghum—I have found that sorghum flour can be difficult to come by in countries outside the United States. Try substituting millet flour in a 1:1 ratio.

Sugar—While sugar is best for creating structure in baked goods, there are a few alternatives. Xylitol can be substituted in a direct 1:1 ratio for sugar, though it will not produce fluffy frostings. Agave may also be substituted, but in order to substitute, lower the baking temperature of the oven by 25 degrees (for example, if the recipe calls for the oven to be at 350°F, then lower it to 325°F); reduce the amount of sweetener by 25 percent (for example, if the recipe calls for 1 cup of sugar, use ³/₄ cup agave); and reduce the amount of liquid in the recipe by 25 percent (for example, if the recipe calls for 1 cup kefir, use ³/₄ cup instead).

Sunflower Seed Butter—Though sunflower seed butter is a great alternative to peanut butter for most people, it doesn't work for everyone. Per 1 cup of sunflower seed butter, you can substitute 1 cup of soy nut butter, or, if you aren't allergic to peanuts, 1 cup of peanut butter.

Measurement Conversions for Cooks outside the United States

The measurements in this book may be confusing to those of you using the metric system. Here is a list of some of the ingredients in this book converted to grams. I have included a couple of other flours that you might use to substitute, as well.

1 cup white rice flour = 98 grams
1 cup Bob's Red Mill Gluten-Free All-Purpose Flour = 151 grams
1 cup garbanzo flour = 115 grams
1 cup potato starch = 174 grams
1 cup granulated sugar = 198 grams
1 cup shortening = 190 grams
1 cup packed dark brown sugar = 240 grams
1 cup packed light brown sugar = 215 grams

There are so many great gluten-free flours on the market, that rather than discuss all of them individually in the substitutions section, I thought it might be more helpful to give you a list of these flours and their weights so that you can substitute them interchangeably. If you are outside the United States, 1 ounce is equal to 28 grams.

1 cup superfine white rice flour = 3.5 ounces
1 cup sorghum flour = 3.9 ounces
1 cup millet flour = 3.9 ounces
1 cup Bob's Red Mill Gluten-Free All-Purpose Flour = 5.4 ounces
1 cup potato starch = 6.2 ounces
1 cup potato flour = 6.2 ounces
1 cup quinoa flour = 3.4 ounces
1 cup garbanzo flour = 4.1 ounces
1 cup tapioca starch = 3.7 ounces
1 cup buckwheat flour = 4.4 ounces

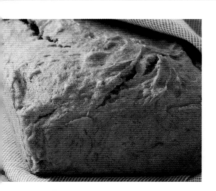
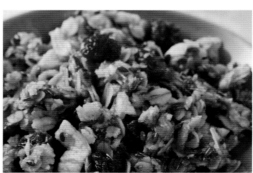
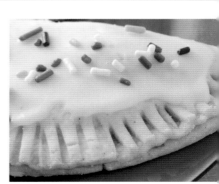

Breakfast Goodies

I love breakfast almost as much as I love dessert, and I have so many fond memories associated with this meal, comforting memories from my childhood. Cinnamon toast and French toast are evocative of the slumber parties of yesteryear, and muffins remind me of bake sales. Sunday morning breakfast or brunch was a time that my entire family came together, and my husband and I have carried on this tradition with our children. We make sure that we either go out or make something together at home every Sunday morning, and the girls have come to count on this practice. Whether you are cooking for yourself, your family, or your friends, I hope that this section will give you plenty of tasty and cozy gluten-, dairy-, soy-, nut- and egg-free ideas.

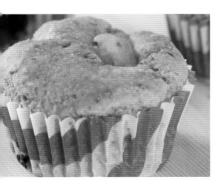
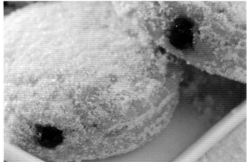
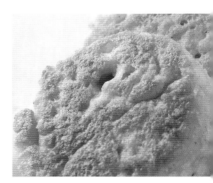

Breakfast Cookies

My daughters are very finicky, but if they know that I have these "cookies" around, getting them to eat breakfast is never a battle. I keep these cookies in the freezer and thaw them as needed so that breakfast takes less than thirty seconds to serve. These little guys are sweet, but they are packed with healthy apples, carrots, gluten-free oats, chunky sunflower seed butter, and bean flour for protein. Best of all, they are completely natural, and the ingredients list is a lot shorter than the one on a box of granola bars. MAKES 48 BREAKFAST COOKIES

2 tablespoons ground flaxseed meal

6 tablespoons water

1½ cups Bob's Red Mill Gluten-Free All-Purpose Baking Flour*

1¾ cups certified gluten-free rolled oats

1 teaspoon baking soda

1 teaspoon baking powder

1 teaspoon xanthan gum

1 cup organic palm fruit oil shortening

¾ cup granulated sugar

¾ cup dark brown sugar

1 cup chunky (or smooth) sunflower seed butter

1 teaspoon vanilla extract

7 ounces apple, shredded

⅓ cup grated carrots

¼ cup shredded coconut

1. Preheat the oven to 350°F. Line two baking sheets with parchment paper and set aside.

2. In a small bowl, combine the flaxseed meal and water and set aside for 3 to 5 minutes. In a large mixing bowl, whisk together the all-purpose baking flour, gluten-free oats, baking soda, baking powder, and xanthan gum. Set aside.

3. In the bowl of a stand mixer, cream together the palm fruit oil shortening, granulated sugar, and brown sugar. Stir in the sunflower seed butter. Scrape down the sides of the bowl and then beat in the flaxseed meal mixture and the vanilla extract. Scrape down the sides again and stir in the flour mixture. Fold in the apple, carrots, and coconut.

4. Using a 1½-inch ice cream scoop, scoop the dough out onto the prepared baking sheets and bake for 16 minutes or until the edges are just golden. Cool completely on the baking sheets. Store leftover cookies in an airtight container for 3 to 5 days.

Note: These cookies freeze well, so I like to freeze most of the completely cooled batch and thaw them overnight in the refrigerator, as needed.

> ✳ If you feel uncomfortable with Bob's products because of possible cross-contamination issues, please see my substitutions guide for ways to work around this product. My substitutions guide provides the weights of common gluten-free flours to make substituting easier.

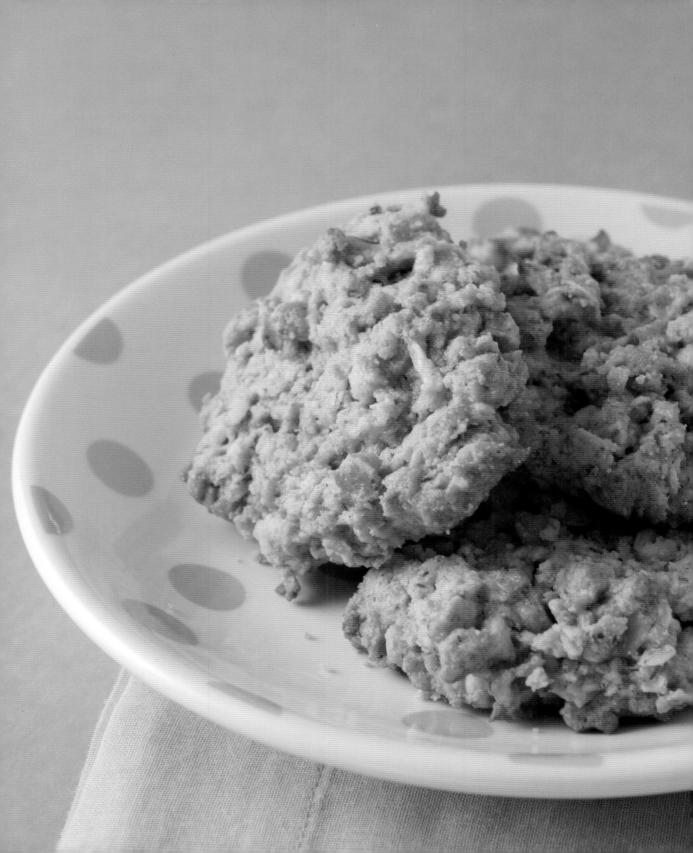

Good Day Granola

Yum, granola. It's just so versatile and crunchy, and I don't know anyone who doesn't love it. Serve it at brunch with a little dairy-free yogurt or milk substitute. Carry a little container of it in your purse for a midmorning snack. However you like to eat granola, making your own at home makes it that much tastier, healthier, and often, lower in fat. SERVES 6

3 cups certified gluten-free
   rolled oats
1 cup whole flaxseeds
1 teaspoon cinnamon
1 teaspoon vanilla extract
$\frac{1}{4}$ cup canola oil
$\frac{1}{4}$ teaspoon salt
$\frac{1}{2}$ cup honey
$\frac{1}{4}$ cup dried apples
$\frac{1}{4}$ cup dried cranberries
$\frac{1}{4}$ cup raisins

1. Preheat the oven to 325°F. Line a rimmed baking sheet with parchment paper and set it aside.

2. In a large bowl combine the oats, flaxseeds, cinnamon, vanilla extract, canola oil, salt, and honey. Dump the mixture out onto the prepared baking sheet. Place the baking sheet in the oven and toast for 30 minutes, stirring every 10 minutes so that it browns evenly.

3. Remove the sheet from the oven and let the mixture cool. Return the cooled oat mixture to the large mixing bowl and add in the dried fruit, tossing to evenly distribute.

4. Store leftover granola in an airtight container, refrigerated, until it is all gone.

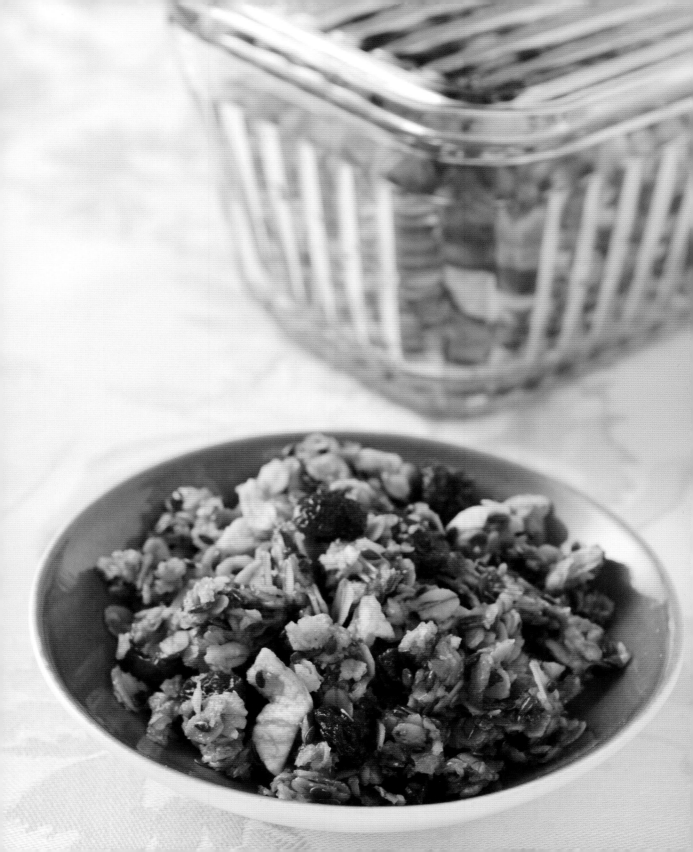

Biscuits

Long before I was diagnosed with food allergies, I spent a few of my teenage years living in Chattanooga, Tennessee. While there I ate Southern biscuits for breakfast nearly every day. Though the method for these biscuits is a bit unorthodox and more like the method for making crumpets, you will be amazed by their lightness and fluffiness. Pull them apart and drizzle them with honey or slather them with jam. Either way they are delicious and so close to the original that you almost won't believe it. MAKES 8 BISCUITS

½ cup plus 3 tablespoons
   warm water
½ teaspoon sugar
1 teaspoon rapid-rise yeast
1 cup Chinese rice flour
⅓ cup potato starch
3 tablespoons plus 1 teaspoon
   sorghum flour
¾ teaspoon salt
1⅛ teaspoons xanthan gum
¾ cup water
1 tablespoon powdered vanilla
   rice milk
1 tablespoon cider vinegar
¾ teaspoon baking soda

1. In a large liquid measuring cup, combine the water and sugar and sprinkle the rapid-rise yeast over the top. Set the yeast aside to proof for 5 to 10 minutes; it should be frothy when you return to it.

2. In a large mixing bowl, whisk together the Chinese rice flour, potato starch, sorghum flour, salt, and xanthan gum. When the yeast and water mixture is ready, pour it into the dry ingredients and mix well. Use your hands, if necessary, to pull the dough into a ball. Cover the dough directly with plastic wrap and then cover the top of the bowl with another sheet of wrap. Place the bowl in a warm place to rise for 45 minutes. The dough will rise but will not double in size.

3. While the dough is rising, mix together the water, powdered rice milk, and cider vinegar. When the dough is ready, pour the baking soda into the water and cider vinegar and immediately pour the mixture over the dough. (It's important that you not add the baking soda until just before mixing the liquid ingredients into the risen dough.) It will seem very wet; I like to use my hands to mix the batter thoroughly. It will be lumpy.

4. Lightly grease a griddle and heat. Meanwhile grease eight 2¾-inch crumpet rings or circular metal pastry cutters. When the griddle is hot, place the greased rings on the griddle and fill each one with about 3 tablespoons of batter. Cook over medium-low heat until they are set, checking the bottoms occasionally to make sure they aren't browning too quickly. If they are browning too quickly, turn down the heat. Cook for about 4 minutes and 30 seconds on the first side. Carefully (they will be hot) remove the rings and flip the biscuits. Cook for another 2 minutes. Remove from the heat and serve warm with jam or honey.

5. The biscuits are best eaten immediately.

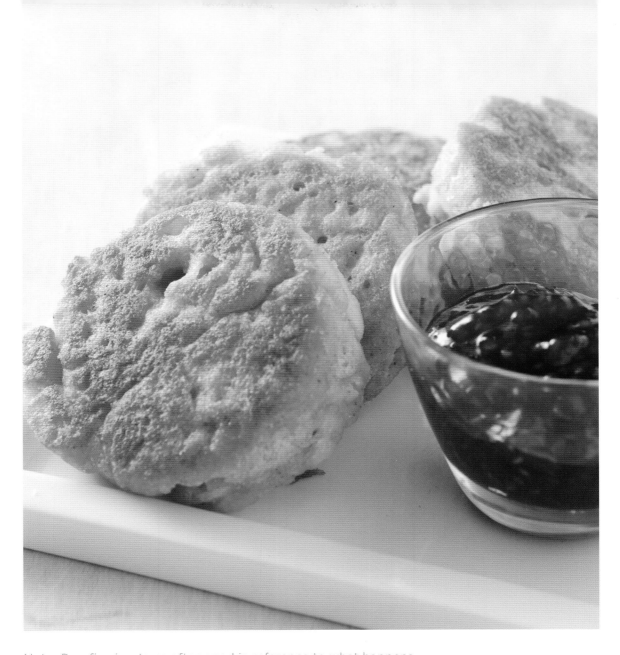

Note: *Proofing* is a term often used in reference to what happens when warm water, yeast, and sugar are mixed and left to sit for a few minutes. After 5 to 10 minutes, the mixture should get frothy, an indication that the yeast is good and that it is activated. If the yeast does not get frothy, then your yeast is old and will not cause your dough to rise. Throw it out and start over with a fresh package.

Stone Fruit Berry Muffins

Everybody loves muffins, but as a mom, I also love to sneak a lot of nutrition into my family's daily diet. Thus when I make muffins, I always load them up with lots of fruit. This way my children feel like they are having cake for breakfast, but I know that they are also getting plenty of vitamins and fiber, too. MAKES 15 MUFFINS

1 cup yellow cornmeal
1 cup sorghum flour
$\frac{1}{2}$ cup sugar
2 teaspoons baking powder
1 teaspoon baking soda
1$\frac{1}{4}$ teaspoons xanthan gum
$\frac{3}{4}$ teaspoon salt
1 tablespoon vanilla rice milk powder
1 cup plain coconut milk kefir
$\frac{1}{2}$ cup unsweetened applesauce
$\frac{1}{4}$ cup canola oil
$\frac{1}{4}$ cup each raspberries, blueberries, diced peaches, and pitted, halved cherries

1. Preheat the oven to 425°F and line 15 muffin tins with paper liners. Set them aside until ready to use.

2. In a large mixing bowl, whisk together the cornmeal, sorghum flour, sugar, baking powder, baking soda, xanthan gum, salt, and vanilla rice milk powder. In a separate, small bowl, stir together the coconut milk kefir, applesauce, and oil. Create a well in the center of the dry ingredients and add the wet ingredients all at once. Stir just until the dry ingredients are moistened. Fold in the fruit.

3. Fill the lined muffin tins $\frac{2}{3}$ of the way full and bake in the preheated oven for 17 minutes or until a toothpick inserted in the center comes out clean.

4. Let the muffins cool for 10 minutes in the tins and then remove them to cooling racks to cool completely. Unused muffins may be stored in an airtight container at room temperature for 3 to 5 days. Completely cooled muffins may be stored, frozen, in an airtight container for up to 3 months.

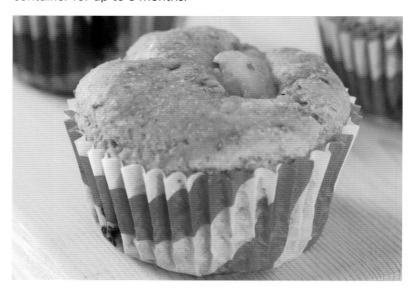

Muesli

What I miss most about my pre-allergic eating is breakfast cereal. Talk about an all-American breakfast. Now, I know that I can get wheat- and egg-free cereals at the supermarket, but all of them are either kind of boring or loaded with sugar. Since I have fond memories of living abroad and eating delicious muesli every day, after finding wheat-free, fruit juice–sweetened cornflakes at the supermarket, I was inspired to make my own gluten-, dairy-, soy-, nut-, and egg-free breakfast cereal. It's delicious with your favorite nondairy milk substitute or yogurt, and it is equally yummy hot or cold. Mix this up once a week and have breakfast for everyone ready in a flash. SERVES 10

1. Pour the gluten-free rolled oats, cornflakes, flaxseed meal, chopped dates, golden raisins, chopped apricots, chopped apples, and pepitas into a large mixing bowl. Using your hands, mix all the ingredients together, breaking up any clumps of dried fruit and making sure that the flaxseed meal is evenly distributed.

2. Scoop the muesli into an airtight container and store, sealed, at room temperature for up to 5 days.

2 1/2 cups gluten-free rolled oats

2 cups gluten-free cornflakes (I prefer the fruit juice–sweetened variety; see Where to Shop section)

1/2 cup ground flaxseed meal

1/2 cup chopped dates

1/2 cup golden raisins

1/4 cup chopped dried apricots

1/4 cup chopped dried apples

1/4 cup pepitas (pumpkin seeds)

Jelly Donuts

Okay, okay, so this isn't exactly the breakfast of champions, but who doesn't love a jelly donut every once in a while? I certainly do. In the summertime, my mother, who was usually fairly strict about eating sweets that she didn't bake at home, often brought jelly donuts for us to have with Sunday brunch. This gluten-, dairy-, soy-, nut-, and egg-free version is absolutely delicious and a terrific addition to any brunch menu. Try serving them for Mardi Gras because they are essentially a gluten-, dairy-, soy-, nut-, and egg-free *paczki.* I always fill mine with a generous squirt of raspberry preserves, but feel free to use any kind of preserves you prefer. **SERVES 11**

¾ cup warmed coconut milk kefir (105°F)

¼ cup warm water (105°F)

1 package dry yeast

¼ cup granulated sugar

½ teaspoon salt

1⅓ cup Chinese or superfine rice flour

1⅓ cup millet flour

1 cup potato starch

½ cup sorghum flour

2½ teaspoons xanthan gum

¼ cup unsweetened applesauce

2 tablespoons canola oil

1 teaspoon vanilla extract

½ cup seltzer water

Canola oil for frying

½ cup raspberry preserves

½ cup granulated sugar

1. Mix together the kefir, water, yeast, sugar, and salt. Set aside to proof for 5 to 10 minutes.

2. Meanwhile, stir together the rice flour, millet flour, potato starch, sorghum flour, and xanthan gum in the bowl of a stand mixer. Add the applesauce, canola oil, and vanilla extract, and mix together to moisten the dry ingredients.

3. Slowly stir in the seltzer and the yeast mixture and then beat them together until a smooth batter forms. Scrape down the sides and then cover the bowl tightly with plastic wrap. Move the bowl to a warm place to rise for 2 hours.

4. When the dough is ready, roll it out on a well-floured surface to a ½-inch thickness, and cut it into eleven 3-inch circles. Loosely cover circles with plastic wrap until the oil is preheated. Fill an electric fryer according to the fryer directions with canola oil and preheat it to 350°F, or heat 3 to 4 inches of oil to 350°F in a large skillet.

5. While the oil is heating, fill a pastry bag fitted with a number 4 tip with the raspberry preserves. Fill a paper bag with ½ cup of granulated sugar.

6. When the oil is ready, place the donuts in the fryer two at a time, frying them for 3 minutes, turning them constantly with tongs, until they are golden. Remove the donuts to paper towels to drain and cool slightly.

7. When the donuts are cool enough to handle, insert the tip of the filled pastry bag about halfway into the side of the donut and fill it with the raspberry preserves until the preserves just barely ooze out of the hole.

8. Place 1 filled donut at a time in the paper bag and very gently shake it to coat the donut. Carefully remove the donut from the bag to a serving tray.

9. Serve immediately. These donuts are best eaten warm.

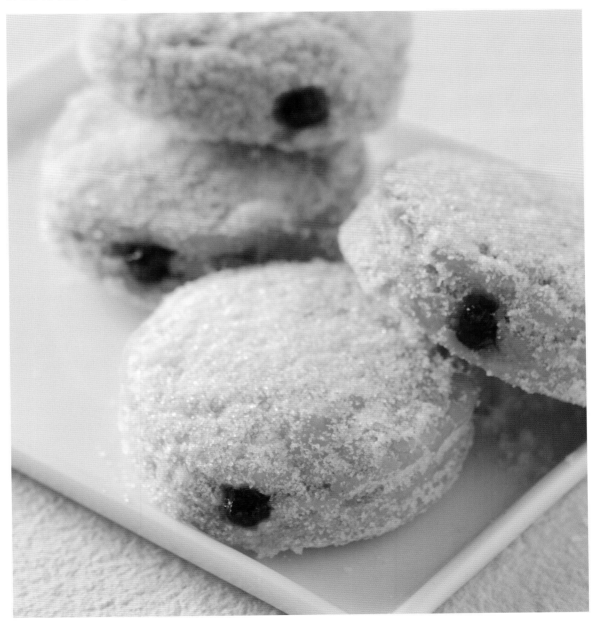

Toaster Turnovers

I remember the first time I tasted a Pop-Tart™. It was the cinnamon-and-brown-sugar flavor, and I thought that it was the best thing that I had ever tasted in my life. I was twelve, and I ate them whenever I babysat for one particular family. My mother never allowed them in our house, so they were a huge treat. I quickly graduated to the strawberry flavor, becoming a devoted fan for many years. Like so many treats, I thought that my wheat and egg allergies spelled the end of my love of the Pop-Tart™. However, I have discovered a way to make my own allergy-free version of the famous toaster pastry. Whatever you do, do not put these in a pop-up toaster. They will burn. You may, however, reheat them for a minute or two on the lowest setting of a toaster oven. MAKES 6 TURNOVERS

1 recipe Basic Double Piecrust
  (page 161)
3 tablespoons strawberry jam
1/4 cup sifted confectioners'
  sugar
1 1/2 teaspoons So Delicious
  original coconut milk, rice
  milk, or water
1/4 teaspoon vanilla extract
Sprinkles or sanding sugar (see
  Where to Shop section)

1. Preheat the oven to 400°F and line a baking sheet with parchment paper.

2. Make the dough according to the recipe instructions and then roll it, between two sheets of parchment paper, into a 13-inch circle, about 1/4 inch thick. Cut the dough with a 5 1/2-inch round cutter and place 1 1/2 teaspoons of the jam on half of each circle. Using a spatula, gently loosen the other side of each turnover and carefully fold it over. If the dough splits when you fold it, moisten your fingers with water and smooth out the crack. Seal the edges with the tines of a fork. Use the spatula to transfer the turnovers to the prepared baking sheet.

3. Bake the turnovers in the preheated oven for 20 minutes or until the edges are just golden brown. Let the turnovers cool on the baking sheet. When they are cool enough to handle, move them to a cooling rack.

4. Make frosting by mixing together the confectioners' sugar, milk substitute of your choice, and vanilla extract. Frost each turnover with a little of the frosting and then sprinkle with sprinkles or sanding sugar.

5. Serve the turnovers warm. These turnovers are best eaten on the day they are made.

> Tip: To cut out these turnovers, I used a lightly-greased cereal bowl rather than a cookie cutter. The bowls were the perfect size.

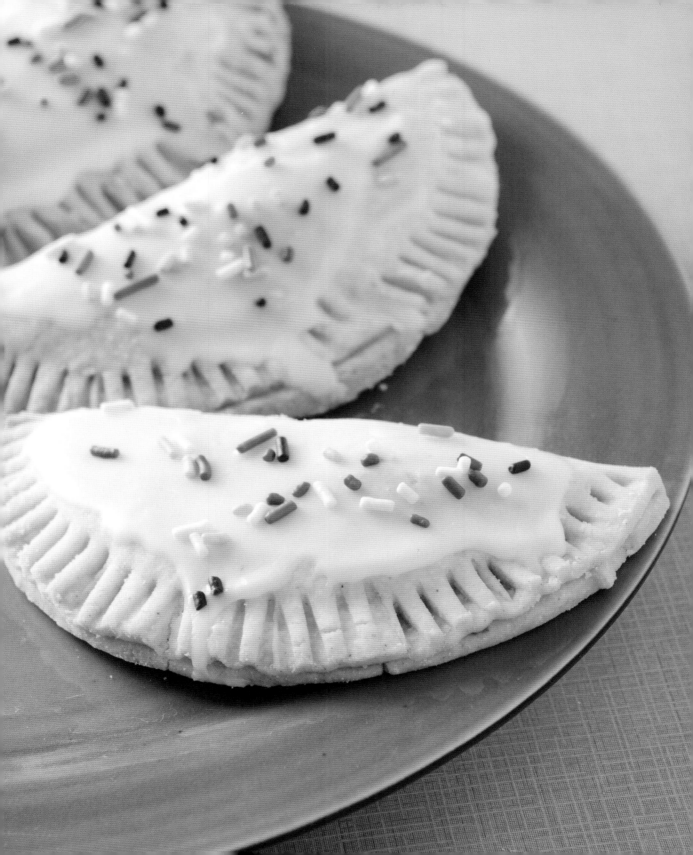

Banana Bread

I know what you're thinking: not another recipe for banana bread! I know that it's such a popular recipe and is in millions of cooking and baking books. However, I chose to include it in this one simply because it's a recipe loved by children nationwide, and it's a great way to use up those last three bananas that are always so dark brown by the end of the week. This is a food that I can always depend on when I need to make a quick breakfast or snack. When banana bread is on their plates, my children never complain, and that is priceless. SERVES 10

1⅓ cups Chinese or superfine rice flour
½ cup potato starch
¼ cup sorghum flour
1 teaspoon cinnamon
1 teaspoon baking powder
1 teaspoon baking soda
1 teaspoon xanthan gum
½ cup organic palm fruit oil shortening
1 cup granulated sugar
½ cup applesauce
3 large, very ripe bananas, mashed
1 tablespoon cider vinegar

1. Preheat the oven to 325°F and lightly grease a 9 x 5-inch loaf pan.

2. In a large bowl whisk together the rice flour, potato starch, sorghum flour, cinnamon, baking powder, baking soda, and xanthan gum; set aside.

3. In the bowl of a stand mixer, cream together the organic palm fruit oil shortening and sugar until light and fluffy. Scrape down the sides and beat in the applesauce and mashed bananas. When the bananas and the applesauce are thoroughly combined, stop the mixer, scrape down the sides again, and beat in the cider vinegar. Slowly stir in the dry ingredients until thoroughly incorporated.

4. Pour the batter into the prepared pan, and bake the banana bread in the preheated oven for 70 minutes or until a toothpick inserted in the center comes out clean. Cool the banana bread in the pan for 15 minutes and then turn out onto a wire rack to cool completely before slicing.

5. Leftovers may be stored tightly wrapped in an airtight container for up to 3 days or frozen tightly wrapped in an airtight container for up to 3 months.

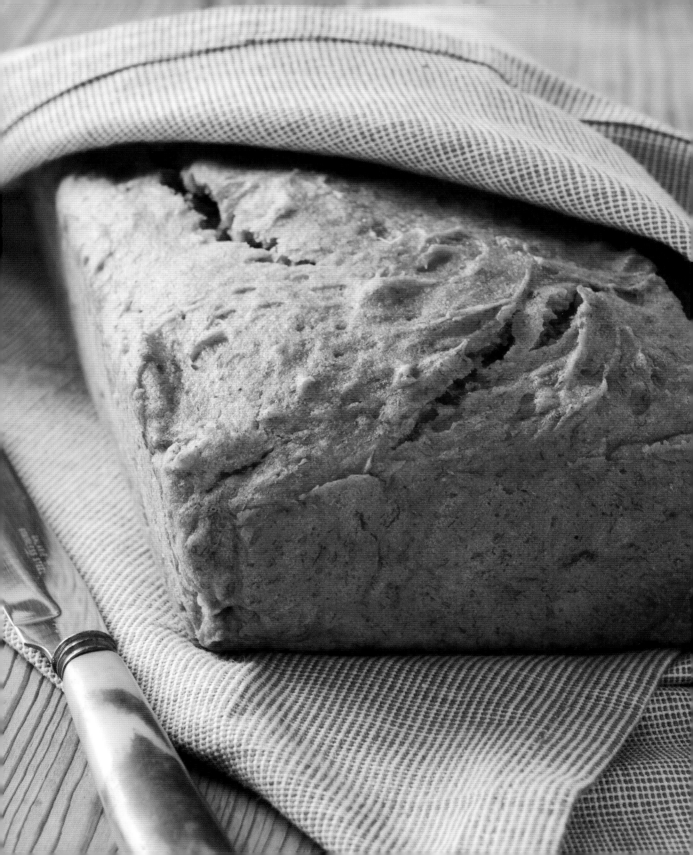

French Toast

French toast was a treat that my mother usually reserved for slumber parties. I always looked forward to Saturday mornings when we got this special, eggy and sweet meal. Until I came up with this recipe one night very recently, I hadn't eaten French toast since 2004. I love the twist of making it with banana bread to give it a little extra something, but you could certainly try making it with my Crusty White Bread (page 136), too. SERVES 4

3 tablespoons flaxseed meal

1 cup So Delicious original
coconut milk or rice milk

½ teaspoon vanilla extract

1 loaf Banana Bread (page 14),
sliced into 10 slices

2 tablespoons canola oil, plus
additional as needed

Maple syrup and sliced
bananas for serving

1. In a large shallow bowl, whisk together the flaxseed meal, coconut or rice milk, and vanilla extract. Let the mixture stand for 3 minutes to thicken.

2. When the flaxseed meal mixture has thickened, carefully lower the slices of banana bread, one at a time, into it on a fork. Coat both sides of the bread with the flaxseed meal mixture.

3. Heat the oil in a large skillet over medium-high heat. Working in batches, fry the coated banana bread in the oil for 3 minutes per side, or until each side is golden brown, adding an additional 1 tablespoon of oil between batches if necessary. Do not flip the bread before 3 minutes or the coating will stick to the pan.

4. Serve the French toast immediately with warm maple syrup and banana slices.

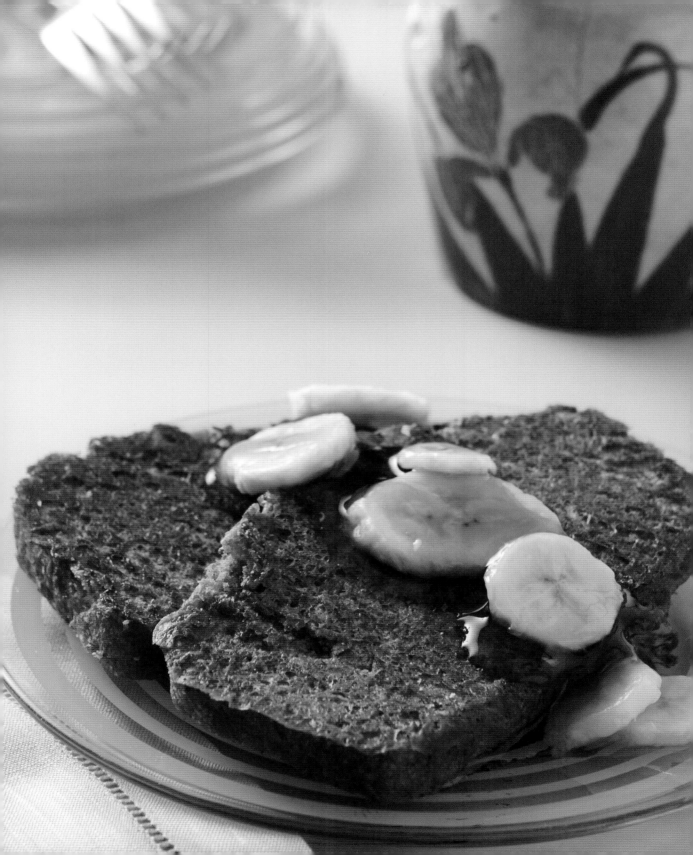

Blueberry Pancakes

The first cookbook that I ever owned was an homage to American heritage and folklore. I was eight or nine when I got it for Christmas. Included in the book were recipes for a Betsy Ross flag cake, Clara Barton bran muffins, and Paul Bunyan and Babe the Blue Ox blueberry pancakes. I made all of these recipes so many times, but my favorite was always the recipe for the pancakes. I felt I couldn't do a comfort food cookbook without one of my very favorite childhood breakfasts. The great thing about this recipe is that you can mix up a batch of the dry mix and keep it in the freezer for whenever the urge to have pancakes moves you. MAKES ABOUT 10–12 SMALL/MEDIUM PANCAKES

Dry Mix

2 cups superfine rice flour
$^2/_3$ cup potato starch
$^1/_3$ cup sorghum flour
$^1/_4$ cup plus 2 tablespoons granulated sugar
2 tablespoons baking powder
1 teaspoon xanthan gum

Pancakes

1$^1/_4$ cups well-whisked dry mix (see above)
$^1/_2$ teaspoon baking soda
1 cup water
1 tablespoon powdered vanilla rice milk
1 tablespoon cider vinegar
1 tablespoon natural applesauce
2 tablespoons canola oil
$^3/_4$ cup fresh blueberries
Confectioners' sugar for dusting
Maple syrup for serving

1. Pour all of the dry mix ingredients into a large airtight container and whisk until thoroughly combined. I like to seal the container and shake it a few times just to be sure it is evenly distributed. Store this dry mix in the freezer to keep the baking powder fresh for up to 3 months.

2. When you are ready to make pancakes, remove the dry mix from the freezer and whisk it again just to be sure the flours didn't settle.

3. To make the pancakes, whisk together the pancake mix and baking soda in a large mixing bowl; set aside.

4. In another bowl combine the water, powdered vanilla rice milk, cider vinegar, and applesauce. When the wet ingredients are well combined, add them, all at once, to the dry ingredients. Whisk until the batter is thoroughly combined and no dry bits remain.

5. Wet a paper towel with a little canola oil and lightly rub the oil on the bottom of a nonstick skillet or griddle. Heat over high heat until a drop of water dances on the griddle or skillet. Turn the heat to medium high and pour the batter into the pan by scant $^1/_4$ cups. Place several blueberries on each pancake. When bubbles in the pancake batter begin to burst, flip the pancakes and cook them through.

6. Remove the pancakes to a plate and serve them dusted with confectioners' sugar and maple syrup. Store completely cooled leftover pancakes that have not been covered with maple syrup with a square of parchment paper between them in an airtight container in the freezer for up to 3 months.

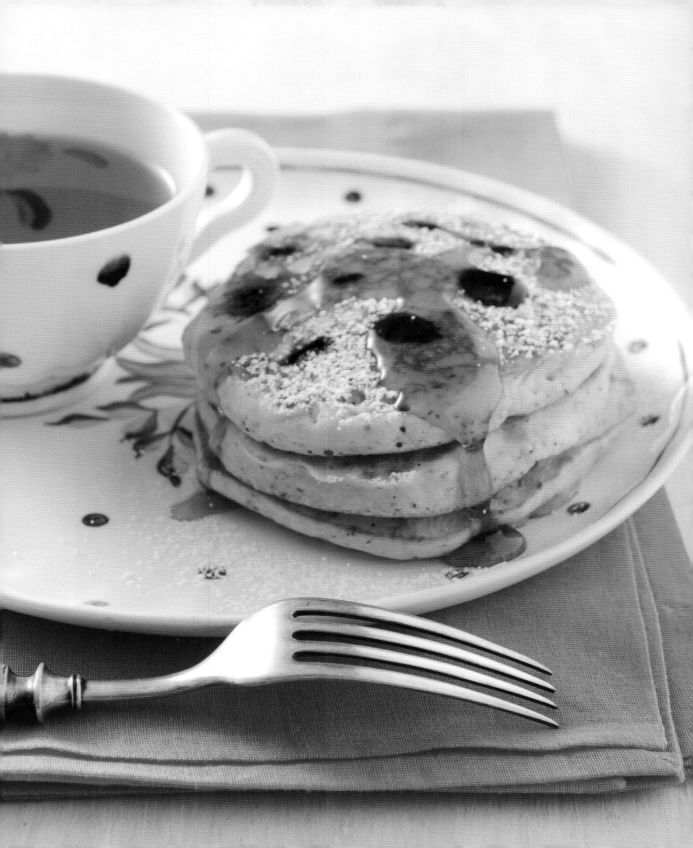

Corned Beef Hash

Corned beef hash is such a staple on New York City diner menus. I can honestly tell you that I've never actually eaten it when I've been out, because I like my version the best. When I was a child, my mother made this with a fried egg on top and called it Hupple Pupple. I have no idea why we called it that, but I can tell you that I requested that meal more than any other when I lived at home. When I learned of my egg allergy, my love affair with Hupple Pupple ended, but I didn't give up the corned beef hash. I love to make it when I have leftover corned beef and potatoes. SERVES 6

2 tablespoons olive oil

¾ cup diced onions

1 pound boiled new potatoes, diced

12 ounces corned beef, finely diced

⅜ teaspoon paprika

¼ teaspoon salt

¼ teaspoon black pepper

1. In a large skillet heat the olive oil over medium-high heat. Add the onions and sauté until soft and translucent, about 3 minutes.

2. Add the potatoes and continue cooking for another 5 minutes or until the potatoes begin to brown.

3. Add the corned beef and paprika, and cook until the potatoes are brown and beginning to crisp and the corned beef is heated through. Add the salt and pepper and serve the hash immediately.

4. Store leftovers, refrigerated, in an airtight container for up to 3 days.

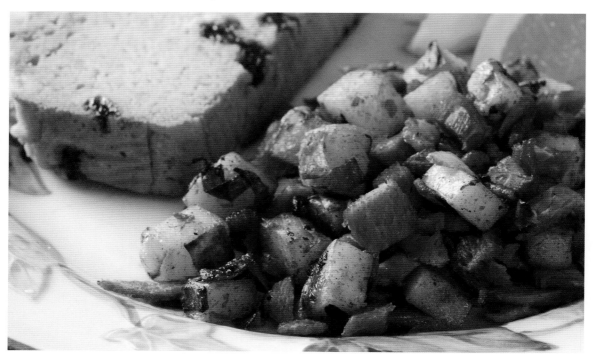

Cinnamon Toast

This was another treat that I had only on the weekends as a child, and I only liked it the way that my mother made it. I loved my mother's method so much so, in fact, that I remember teaching a friend's mother how to make it under the broiler instead of in the toaster. I'm sure she was thrilled. However, cinnamon toast just isn't the same when the bread is toasted first. The middle of the bread doesn't get as soft nor the topping as gooey. When making cinnamon toast this way, just be sure to keep your eye on it when it is under the broiler. It can burn in a flash. MAKES 10 SLICES OF CINNAMON TOAST

1. Preheat the broiler.

2. In a small bowl mix together the sugar and cinnamon until evenly combined.

3. Spread each slice of bread with 1 teaspoon of the margarine and then place on an unlined baking sheet.

4. Using a spoon, sprinkle the cinnamon-sugar mixture over the "buttered" slices of bread. You may not need all of the cinnamon-sugar mixture to cover the bread; use as much or as little as you desire.

5. Place the prepared bread under the broiler for 30 to 45 seconds, watching it the entire time to be sure it doesn't burn. The cinnamon toast is finished when the margarine and sugar are melted and the edges are just golden. Serve immediately.

$1/4$ cup granulated sugar
2 teaspoons cinnamon
1 loaf Crusty White Bread (page 136), sliced into 10 slices
10 teaspoons dairy- and soy-free margarine

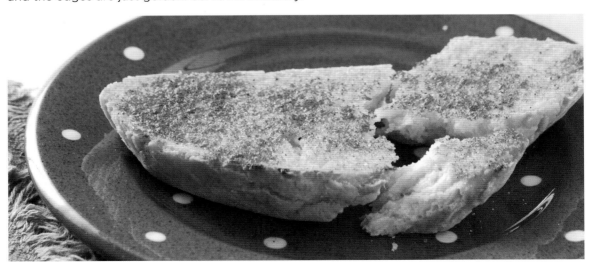

Funnel Cakes

These are a very special brunch treat, and something that I make only occasionally. They are, however, a showstopper and therefore very fun to serve at a casual holiday brunch or a lazy summer brunch. Funnel cakes are something that we ate just once a year in Ohio, because you could only get them at the fair. They were also one of the very first things we learned how to make in eighth-grade Home Ec, so I still think of my teacher every time I make them. MAKES ABOUT 4-6 CAKES

Canola oil for frying
1 tablespoon cider vinegar
2 tablespoons powdered vanilla rice milk
2 cups water
2 tablespoons applesauce
1 teaspoon vanilla extract
2 cups Arrowhead Mills All-Purpose Baking and Pancake Mix
1 teaspoon xanthan gum
1 teaspoon baking soda
$\frac{1}{2}$ teaspoon salt
1 tablespoon sugar
$\frac{1}{4}$ cup canola oil
Confectioners' sugar for dusting

1. Fill a fryer with canola oil according to the fryer instructions, or fill a large skillet with 3 to 4 inches of canola oil. Preheat the fryer or pan to 350°F.

2. While the oil is preheating, whisk together the vinegar, vanilla rice milk powder, water, applesauce, and vanilla extract in a large bowl; set aside.

3. In the bowl of a stand mixer, stir together the baking mix, xanthan gum, baking soda, salt, and sugar until well combined. Beat in the wet ingredients and then stir in the $\frac{1}{4}$ cup of canola oil until it is combined.

4. Pour the batter into a large funnel with your finger over the spout to keep it from spilling out. When the oil is hot enough, release your finger from the bottom of the funnel and let the batter run out, moving the funnel around so that the cakes are vaguely spiral in shape. Fry the funnel cake for about 3 to 4 minutes per side or until the cake is golden brown on both sides.

5. Remove the funnel cake from the oil with a metal slotted spatula and drain on paper towels. Repeat until you have used all the batter. Dust the drained funnel cakes with confectioners' sugar and serve immediately while warm.

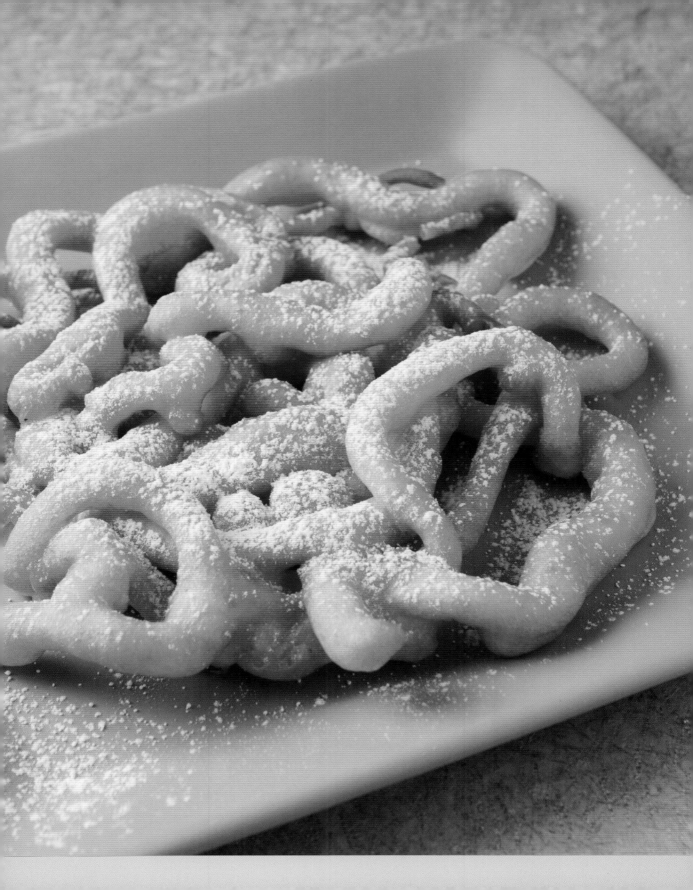

Pot Stickers

Even growing up in small town Ohio, there was a Chinese restaurant, and we all clamored for pan-fried pork dumplings. So, for me, this dish is definitely a favorite. Not to mention the fact that this is one of the few dishes that all four of my family members will gobble up without complaint. While I loved the fried pork version when I was younger, I much prefer the vegetarian version today. **MAKES 26 POT STICKERS**

1⅓ cups Chinese or superfine rice flour

½ cup potato starch

¼ cup sorghum flour

1¾ teaspoons xanthan gum

¼ teaspoon salt

⅔ cup organic palm fruit oil shortening

½ cup cold water

2 tablespoons canola oil, divided, plus additional if needed

2 garlic cloves, minced

1 cup (about ¼ pound) diced shiitake mushrooms

1½ teaspoons minced ginger root

1 very small head Napa cabbage, shredded (about 4 cups)

3 scallions, white and light green parts only, thinly sliced

1 tablespoon rice wine (mirin)

¼ teaspoon sesame oil (optional)

1 cup water

1. Place the rice flour, potato starch, sorghum, xanthan gum, and salt in the bowl of a food processor and pulse once or twice just to blend them. Add the organic palm fruit oil shortening and pulse until pea-size chunks form. Add the cold water and pulse again until a dough forms. Gather the dough into a ball and wrap it tightly in plastic wrap until you are ready to use it.

2. To make the filling, heat 1 tablespoon of the canola oil in a large frying pan over medium-high heat and sauté the garlic until it begins to soften, about 1 to 2 minutes. Add in the mushrooms and ginger and continue cooking until the mushrooms have shrunk in size and the ginger has softened. Add in the Napa cabbage, scallions, rice wine, and sesame oil. Continue cooking until the filling has reduced in size to about half and the cabbage is nice and soft; remove from the heat.

3. Roll out the dough on a well-floured surface to ⅛-inch thickness and cut it with a 2½-inch round cutter. Cover the cut dough with a piece of plastic wrap to keep it from drying as you work on each dumpling. Fill each round with 1½ teaspoons of filling and then pinch the edges together with your fingers. Place the finished dumplings on a rimmed baking sheet and cover with a damp cloth to keep them from drying out as you work.

4. When all the dumplings have been filled, heat the remaining tablespoon of canola oil over medium-high heat in a large nonstick skillet fitted with a lid. When the oil is hot, add as many dumplings as will fit in the pan, but do not overcrowd them. Brown the dumplings on both sides, about 2 minutes per side. When all the dumplings are browned on both sides, add 1 cup of water to the pan and quickly cover the pan. Turn up the heat to high, and steam the dumplings for 5 minutes. Do not lift the lid.

5. Remove the steamed dumplings to a platter and loosely tent with tin foil while you make additional batches of the dumplings, adding an additional 1 tablespoon of canola oil to the pan for the frying between batches, if necessary. Serve the dumplings immediately.

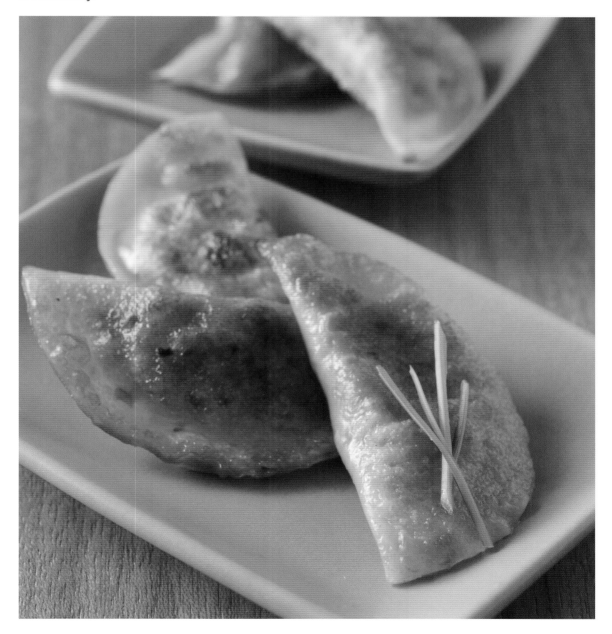

Italian Wedding Soup

One day I was strolling through the supermarket aisles just sort of daydreaming when my eyes fell upon a can of this soup. It brought me back to when one of my cousins married a very Italian girl, and we actually had Italian wedding soup as a starter at their wedding reception. A sucker for meatballs even at eleven years old, I thought this was the most glamorous and exotic dish I had ever tasted. I hadn't had it for many years because the meatballs usually contain eggs and wheat, but now I eat it about once a week. SERVES 6–8

½ pound chicken
1 tablespoon Italian parsley
¾ teaspoon salt
Dash pepper
1 clove garlic, pressed
1 teaspoon cornstarch
1 tablespoon plus 2 teaspoons olive oil, divided
½ cup diced onions
½ cup sliced carrots
½ cup diced celery
6 cups Chicken Stock (page 112)

1. Place the chicken, parsley, salt, pepper, clove of garlic, and cornstarch in the bowl of a food processor and pulse until the chicken is finely minced and all the ingredients are combined. Using a measuring spoon, scoop teaspoonfuls of the meat and roll into little meatballs. Heat 1 teaspoon of the olive oil over high heat in a large skillet. Place the meatballs in the heated oil and brown on all sides.

2. While the meatballs are browning, heat the remaining oil over medium-high heat in a large pot and sauté the onions, sliced carrots, and diced celery until they begin to soften and the onion is translucent.

3. When the vegetables are soft, add the stock and meatballs and bring the soup to a boil. When the soup reaches a full boil, turn down the heat to a simmer and simmer for 5 minutes or until the meatballs are cooked through. Adjust the salt and pepper, if necessary, before serving.

4. Leftovers may be stored in airtight containers, refrigerated, for up to 3 days. The completely cooled soup may also be frozen in airtight containers for up to 3 months.

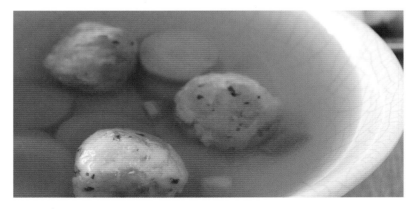

Vegetarian Vegetable Soup

Someone once told me that your plate should be three-quarters vegetables and one-quarter everything else. I like to serve this vegetable soup as a starter or main course to accomplish that ratio. I make up big batches and keep it in the fridge for a quick lunch, or I serve it as a first course when we are having friends over for dinner. Everyone needs to eat more vegetables, and I find it much easier to do so when the vegetables come in the form of a warm and hearty vegetable soup.

SERVES 8

1. Heat the olive oil in a large stockpot over medium-high heat. Add the onion and garlic and sauté until they begin to soften, about 2 to 3 minutes.

2. Add the carrots, zucchini, and celery and cook until the vegetables begin to soften, about 8 minutes.

3. Stir in the salt, Italian seasoning, dried parsley, and red pepper flakes, if using. Pour in the diced tomatoes and add the cannellini beans, stock, and kale. Bring the soup to a full boil and then reduce to a simmer. Simmer for 10 minutes. Stir in the black pepper and serve.

4. Leftovers may be kept in airtight containers, refrigerated, for up to 3 days, or the soup may be frozen in airtight containers for up to 3 months.

2 tablespoons olive oil
1 medium onion, diced (about 1 cup)
1 clove garlic, minced
2 medium carrots, diced (about 2 cups)
2 medium zucchini, diced (about 2 cups)
1 celery stalk, diced
1½ teaspoons salt
1 teaspoon Italian seasoning
½ teaspoon dried parsley flakes
¼ teaspoon red pepper flakes (optional)
1 28-ounce can diced tomatoes with their juice
1 19-ounce can cannellini beans, rinsed and drained
3 cups vegetable or Chicken Stock (page 112)
1 cup chopped kale, stems removed
½ teaspoon black pepper

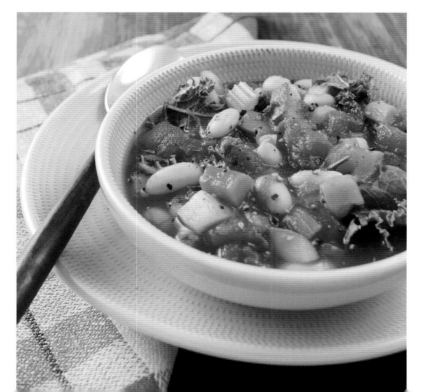

Dolmades

I love dolmades, and they are almost always served with Greek salads at New York City diners. Also served as an appetizer, they make people think you slaved in the kitchen, but really they don't take more than thirty minutes to make and only taste better the longer they steep in their own herbs. Our family loves them, and I like to keep extras on hand for a snack with a little bit of hummus. MAKES 26 DOLMADES

1 cup Chicken Stock (page 112)
2 cups water
⅓ cup olive oil
¼ cup diced onions
2 garlic cloves, minced
¾ cup Arborio rice
⅓ cup chopped mint
⅓ cup chopped fresh dill
¼ cup lemon juice (from about 1 lemon)
¼ teaspoon salt
26–39 jarred cooked grape leaves (about 1 15-ounce jar)

1. Heat the chicken stock and water in a saucepan to a simmer. Turn the heat to the very lowest setting.

2. While the water and stock are heating, heat the olive oil in a large skillet over medium-high heat. Add the onions and minced garlic and sauté until they are translucent and fragrant, about 3 to 4 minutes.

3. Add the Arborio rice and stir to coat it with the oil. Cook for 1 minute to open the rice grains. Add 2 cups of the water and stock to the rice and stir. The stock should immediately boil. Turn the heat down to medium. Stir the rice until all of the water is absorbed, repeating the process of adding water and stirring until the rice is tender and creamy. When all of the stock and water have been added and absorbed, remove the rice from the heat.

4. Stir in the mint, dill, lemon juice, and salt.

5. Drain the grape leaves and remove the roll from the jar. Depending on the desired size of the dolmades and the condition of the leaves (sometimes they are torn), place 1 to 2 leaves on a flat working surface. Spoon 1 tablespoon of the rice filling into the center of the leaf or leaves. Fold in three of the sides to create an envelope and then roll up the dolmades. Place the dolmades seam side down on a serving plate or in a storage container.

6. The dolmades may be served immediately, warm, or stored in the refrigerator in an airtight container for 3 to 5 days. They are also delicious cold.

Corn Chowder

The corn out on Long Island is so delicious in July and August that I like to buy extra, steam it, cut the corn off the cob, and freeze it so that I can make things like this corn chowder all year long. This is one of my husband's favorites. Serve it as a first course or with a few slices of Crusty White Bread (page 186) for a light winter lunch. SERVES 8

1. Place the potatoes in a large pot and cover with water. Bring them to a boil and boil for about 15 minutes or until they are fork tender. Drain the potatoes and set aside.

2. Meanwhile, cook the bacon in a large stockpot over medium heat until crisp, about 10 minutes. With a slotted spoon, remove the bacon to a paper towel–lined plate to drain.

3. Cook the diced onion in the remaining bacon fat; sauté until it is soft and translucent, about 5 minutes.

4. Add the stock, coconut milk, corn, salt, black pepper, thyme, and potatoes to the stockpot. Bring the soup to a simmer and let it simmer for 10 minutes. Do not boil. Stir in the bacon. Serve while hot.

5. Store leftovers in airtight containers, refrigerated, for up to 3 days. The completely cooled soup may also be frozen in airtight containers for up to 3 months.

Note: If you have frozen this soup and worry when you take it out of the freezer about the clotted coconut milk, never fear, it will return to its liquid state when it is gently warmed.

½ pound new potatoes, scrubbed and quartered

3 slices soy-free bacon, chopped

1 small onion, diced

1 cup Chicken Stock (page 112)

3 cups So Delicious original coconut milk

10 ounces (about 1½ cups) corn (fresh or frozen)

¾ teaspoon salt

¼ teaspoon black pepper

⅛ teaspoon dried thyme

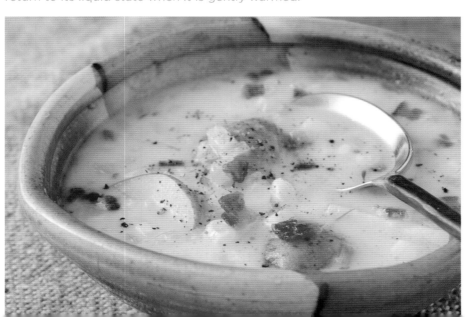

Buffalo Wings

My husband loves buffalo wings, and his eyes lit up when I said that I was including a gluten-, dairy-, soy-, nut-, and egg-free recipe for them in this book. He started a diet just before I started testing recipes, so I had to bake these for him. We discovered that they taste great baked or fried! You can either fry or bake these depending on your dietary needs. They are crispier when fried but equally delicious when baked. Despite his diet, my husband wolfed down quite a few as he watched a winter football game. SERVES 5

20 chicken wings
1 recipe All-Purpose Breading
  (page 66)
1¼ cup rice milk
¾ cup Frank's Red Hot
  Cayenne Pepper Sauce
3 tablespoons canola oil, plus
  additional for misting (see
  Where to Shop guide)
Ranch Dressing (page 64) and
  celery sticks for serving

1. With poultry shears or a very sharp knife, cut off the tips of the chicken wings and then cut the wings in half at the joint.

2. Lightly grease two rimmed baking sheets and set them aside.

3. Make the All-Purpose Breading according to the recipe instructions and pour it into a large, shallow bowl.

4. Pour the rice milk into a separate bowl. Dip each wing into the rice milk and then into the breading. Place the breaded wings on the prepared baking sheets, cover them, and refrigerate for 1 hour.

5. When the wings have chilled, preheat the oven to 400°F. Remove the wings from the refrigerator and lightly mist them with some canola oil. Bake the wings for 45 to 50 minutes, flipping them halfway through, or until the juices run clear when they are poked with a knife and they are golden brown.

6. While the wings are baking, stir together the hot sauce and canola oil and set it aside.

7. Remove the wings from the oven and pour the sauce over them, carefully turning the wings with tongs, so as not to knock off the breading, in order to thoroughly coat them with the sauce. Serve them immediately with celery sticks and Ranch Dressing.

> Tip: To fry the wings, heat the fryer to 350°F while the wings are chilling. Remove the chilled wings from the refrigerator and fry them several at a time, being careful not to overcrowd the fryer, for about 7 minutes. Remove them to paper towels to drain, then place them on a rimmed baking sheet, and cover with sauce. Serve immediately.

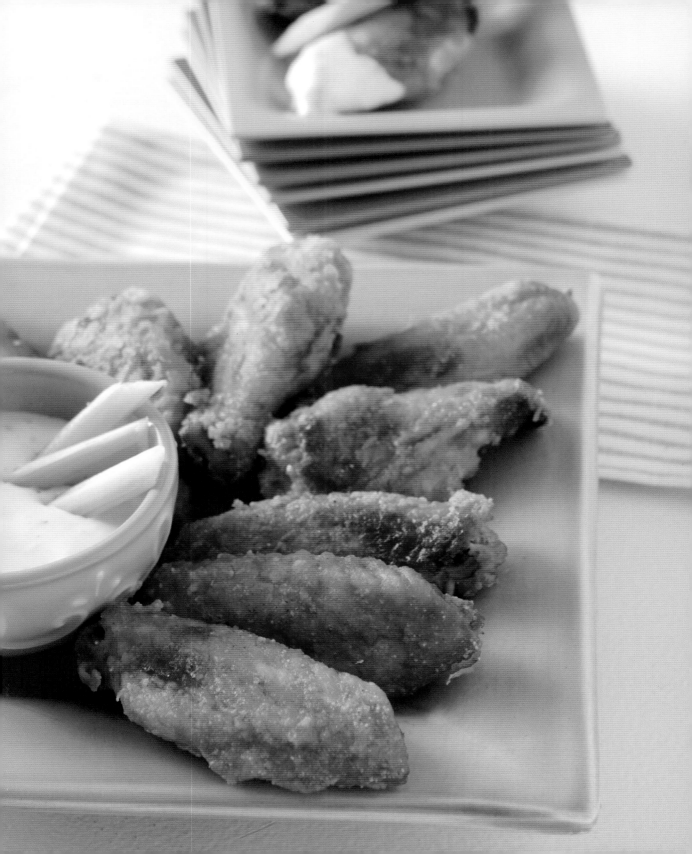

Bacon-Wrapped Dates

Without fail I make these when I need to bring an appetizer to a party or want to have a little finger food out at a party at our house. Everyone loves the savory and sweet combination, and therefore they are always a hit. I love them because they take all of five minutes to construct and I can pop them in the oven just before I walk out the door or the guests walk in. After the first time I made these, they became a permanent fixture on our family's Thanksgiving menu. SERVES 10

20 pitted Medjool dates
7 slices soy-free bacon
Toothpicks

1. Preheat the oven to 400°F.

2. Starting at the end of 1 slice of bacon, wrap 1 date until it is just covered with bacon. Cut the bacon with a sharp knife and then poke a toothpick through the bacon and the date vertically to hold it together. Place the wrapped date on a baking sheet. Repeat the process until all of the dates are wrapped.

3. Place the dates in the oven and bake for 6 minutes. Turn the dates over and continue baking for another 6 minutes. Serve immediately for maximum crispiness.

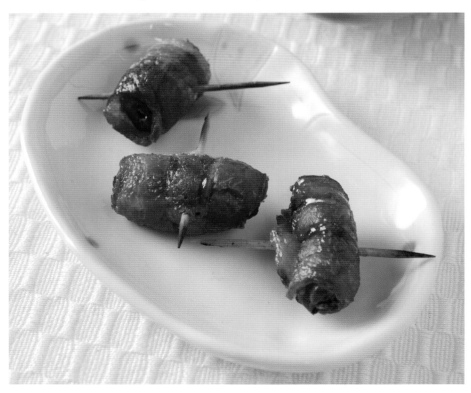

Curried Pumpkin Seeds

When I lived in France, I could always count on cashews, olives, and a kir to get the evening started—a little light snack before dinner. However, with so many people allergic to peanuts and tree nuts, I thought it would be interesting to include something as salty and crunchy as cashews, but safe for those of us with food allergies. Snack away! SERVES 10

1. In a large mixing bowl, combine the canola oil, curry powder, cayenne pepper, and salt; set aside.

2. Heat a large skillet over medium-high heat. Add the pumpkin seeds and toast them until the pumpkin seeds begin to puff slightly and become just golden brown, about 4 minutes.

3. Toss the toasted pumpkin seeds with the canola oil and spice mix and serve warm or at room temperature.

4. Store uneaten pumpkin seeds in an airtight container for up to 3 days.

1 tablespoon plus 1 teaspoon canola oil
3 teaspoons Madras curry powder
⅛ teaspoon cayenne pepper powder
1 teaspoon coarse sea salt
2 cups raw pumpkin seeds

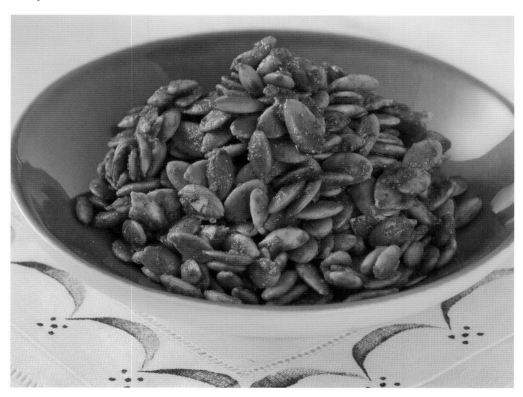

Pigs in a Blanket

These little yummies are ubiquitous on the cocktail party circuit. I like to serve them at kids' parties instead of giant hot dogs that I know will end up getting thrown away. A pig in a blanket is just the right size for little hands and little tummies. Serve them with a little Dijon mustard, ketchup, or BBQ Sauce (page 61) for dipping. MAKES 55

1 recipe All-Purpose Savory
   Pastry (page 67)
19 gluten-, dairy-, soy-, nut-,
   and egg-free hot dogs, cut
   into thirds

1. Preheat the oven to 400°F and prepare the All-Purpose Savory Pastry dough according to the recipe directions.

2. On a well-floured surface, roll the pastry dough into a large rectangle, about 24 x 18 inches. Square off the sides with a knife. Cut the rectangle into $2^3/_4$ x 3-inch strips.

3. Place a third of a hot dog at the end of one of the strips and roll up the dog. Gently press the seams together so that the blanket stays closed.

4. Place the pigs in a blanket on an ungreased rimmed baking sheet and cover with a damp cloth as you continue rolling the other hot dogs. Continue rolling the hot dogs and then re-rolling the dough and cutting it into strips until all of the hot dogs have been wrapped.

5. Bake the pigs in a blanket in the preheated oven for 12 minutes. Serve immediately with Dijon mustard, BBQ Sauce (page 61), or ketchup for dipping.

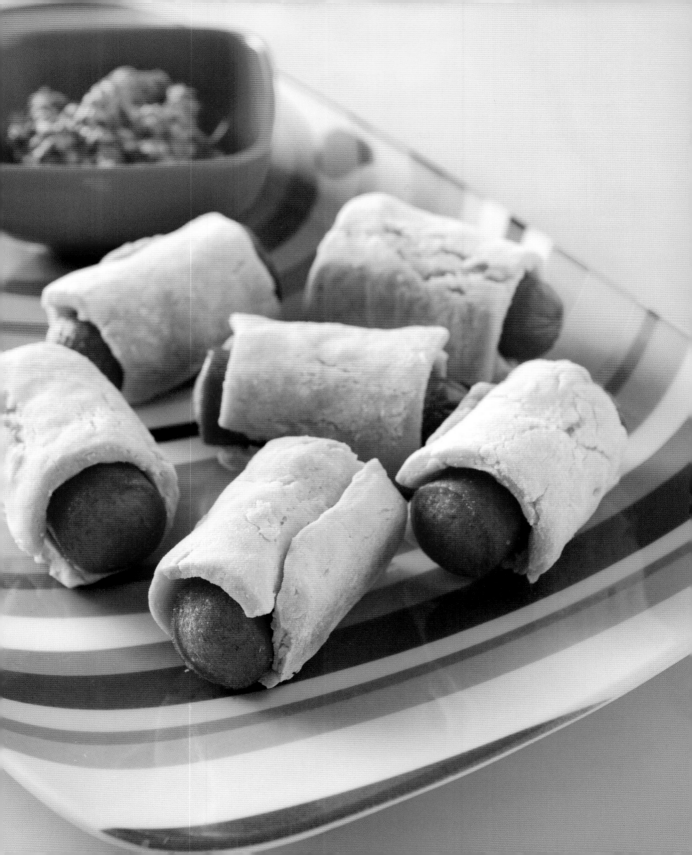

Nachos

Call me a snob, but I really prefer nachos when they are made with warm homemade chips. This way I also know that the chips have not come into contact with any wheat. Be careful when you are making these that you read the corn tortilla ingredients. Some corn tortillas are still made with wheat. These are so fun to serve for the big game when friends are over to help gobble them up.
SERVES 8

Canola oil for frying
20 6-inch corn tortillas, each
    cut into 6 pieces
1 teaspoon salt, divided
1 cup Weeknight Turkey Chili
    (page 97)
1 cup Daiya cheese or your
    favorite allergy-friendly
    cheese (optional)
½ avocado, cubed
2 scallions chopped
¼ cup canned jalapeño
    peppers, chopped (optional)

1. Fill a fryer with canola oil according to the fryer instructions or fill a large skillet with 3 to 4 inches of canola oil. Preheat the fryer or the oil in the skillet to 350°F. Working in 4 batches so as not to overcrowd the fryer, fry the tortilla pieces for about 2 minutes. Remove the chips from the fryer to a paper towel–lined baking sheet to drain. Sprinkle each batch with ¼ teaspoon salt.

2. When all of the tortilla chips have been cooked and are cool enough to handle, pile them on a large platter. If the chili is left-over, warm it up for 2 minutes, covered, in the microwave. Then add it to the top of the nachos.

3. If you are using a cheese substitute, sprinkle it on top. If the cheese does not melt on top of the warm chili, heat the nachos under the broiler for another 30 seconds, watching them constantly to ensure that the cheese does not burn.

4. Add the avocado to the top of the nachos and sprinkle them with the scallions and the jalapeños (if using). Serve immediately.

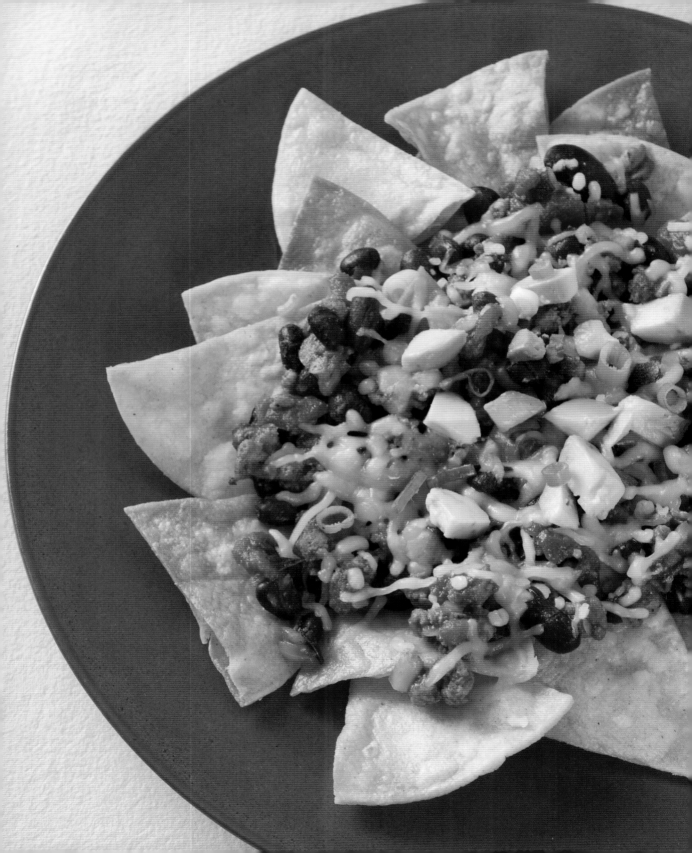

White Bean and Rosemary Hummus

Whenever I ask people to name their favorite side to bring to a potluck, they consistently respond: "Hummus." I agree. It's easy, healthy, delicious, and, for the most part, kids and adults alike enjoy it. However, sometimes I just need a change of pace, and just by changing two of the ingredients, I can achieve a subtle, but lovely difference. This hummus is especially tasty served with the homemade corn chips from my nachos recipe (page 38) or crudités, and it's as simple to make as the original. MAKES 1⅓ CUPS

1 19-ounce can cannellini
    beans, drained, and 1
    tablespoon of liquid
    reserved
1 clove garlic
¼ teaspoon salt
1¼ teaspoons chopped fresh
    rosemary
2 teaspoons lemon juice
¼ cup olive oil
Corn tortilla chips or crudités
    for serving

1. Place the cannellini beans, garlic, salt, rosemary, and lemon juice in the bowl of a food processor, and process until smooth but thick.

2. With the food processor on, pour in the olive oil in a slow and steady stream. Continue processing and add the reserved bean liquid with the motor running. Process just until the liquid is mixed in and the hummus is smooth.

3. Serve immediately with chips or vegetables. Leftovers may be stored in an airtight container, refrigerated, for up to 3 days.

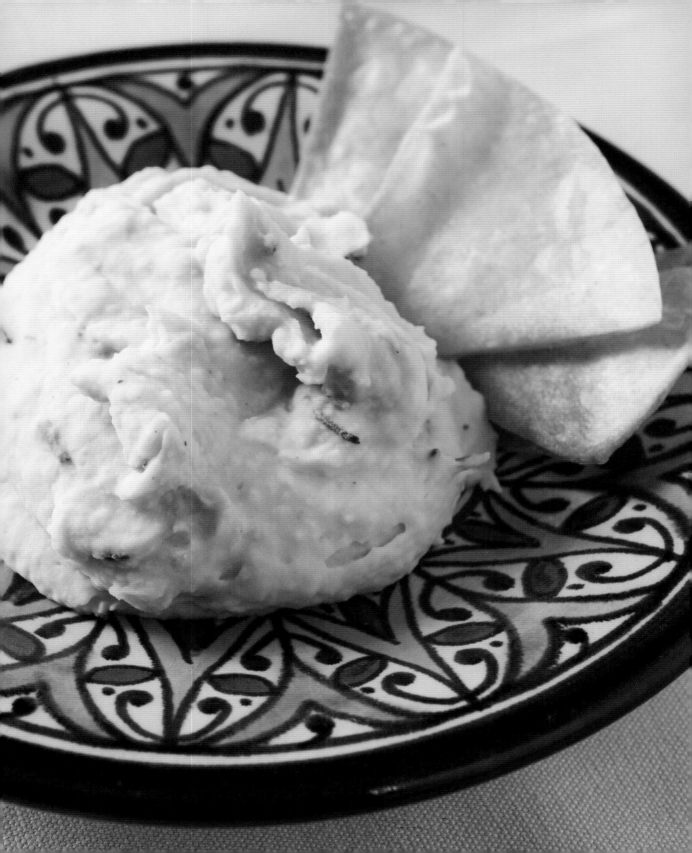

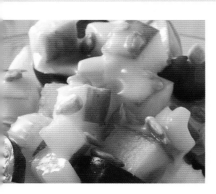
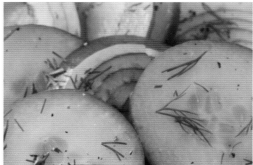
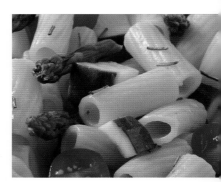

Salads

When I *think* of salad, an image of limp lettuce on a plate with tomato wedges and slices of onion comes to mind. I'm not a big fan. However, when I *make* a salad, it is a completely different story. I like salads that could be the centerpiece of the meal, and I love hearty salads filled with various colors and flavors. Sometimes I make giant lettuce-based salads, but in this book, I wanted to do classic, comfort food salads like potato salad and Waldorf salad, dishes that have a special place in many of our hearts but that food allergies have eliminated from our diets. On the following pages you will find many terrific side salads that are big on flavor but remain gluten, dairy, soy, nut, and egg free.

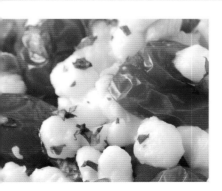 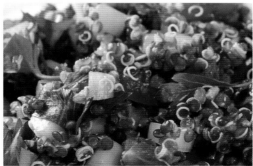 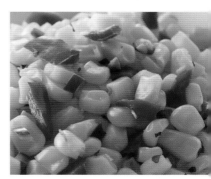

Potato Salad

What is a picnic without potato salad? I can't remember a single Memorial Day or Fourth of July get-together of yesteryear that didn't include potato salad. I used to love my mom's recipe, but unfortunately hers includes both hard-boiled eggs and mayonnaise. I decided to use a light Dijon vinaigrette to both lighten up my recipe and to make it gluten, dairy, soy, nut, and egg free. My family loves this potato salad so much that we don't just eat it in the summer; we enjoy it all year long. SERVES 6

2 pounds Yukon Gold potatoes, scrubbed and quartered

Salt to taste

1 bunch scallions, white and light green parts only, thinly sliced

3 ribs celery, sliced

1 recipe Traditional Dijon Vinaigrette (page 60)

3 slices soy-free bacon, cooked crisp

1. Place the potatoes in a large pot and cover with water and a generous pinch of salt. Bring the water to a boil and boil the potatoes for 20 minutes or until they are soft. Remove the potatoes from the heat and drain.

2. Place the drained potatoes in a large serving bowl. Add in the sliced scallions and celery and combine. I like to use my hands to thoroughly incorporate all the ingredients.

3. Pour the vinaigrette over the top and combine with a wooden spoon. Crumble the bacon over the top, toss gently, and cover the bowl with plastic wrap.

4. Place the bowl in the refrigerator for at least an hour before serving to let the flavors ripen and the potatoes cool. I like to make this the night before so it has plenty of time for all the flavors to intensify. Taste the salad and add a pinch of salt if necessary.

5. Store leftovers in an airtight container, in the refrigerator, for up to 5 days.

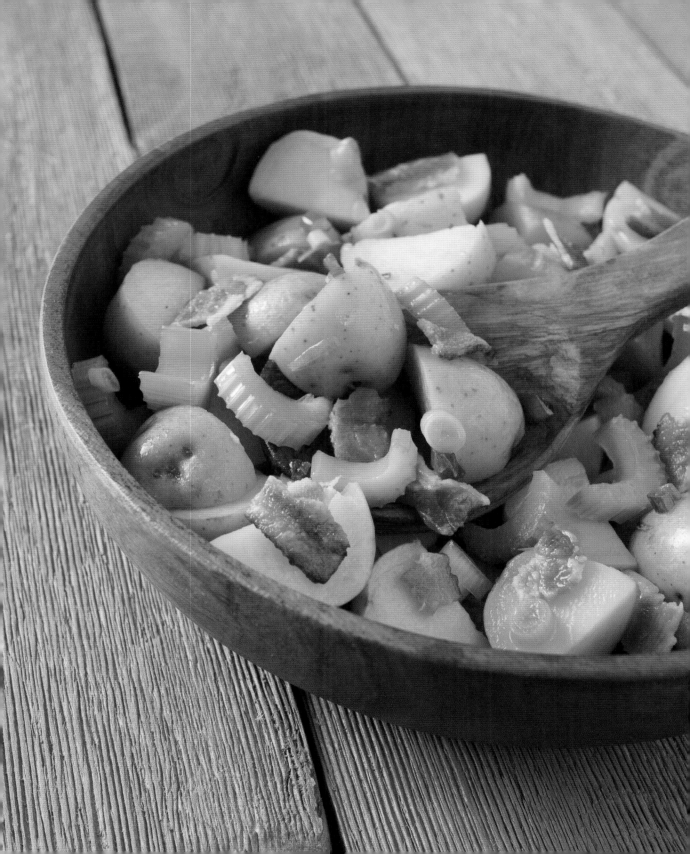

Avocado Salad

I have learned that some of the most impressive dishes are the simplest, styled to beauty. Half of the joy of eating is the visual experience of the dish. I always scoop out the avocados in this salad with a melon baller. Trust me: Something so easy makes people go gaga. Neither you nor your guests will be disappointed by this simple side salad. SERVES 8–10

4 ripe avocados, scooped into balls with a melon baller

1 small tomato, seeded and diced

3 tablespoons lime juice

½ teaspoon cumin

1 teaspoon salt

1 bunch scallions, very thinly sliced

1 tablespoon finely chopped cilantro

1. Layer the avocados and tomatoes in a large serving bowl.

2. Mix together the lime juice, cumin, and salt. Pour the dressing over the avocados and tomatoes.

3. Sprinkle the salad first with the scallions and then with the cilantro. Serve immediately.

4. Leftovers may be stored, refrigerated with plastic wrap pressed directly on top, in an airtight container for up to 2 days, but the avocados may brown.

Waldorf Salad

When I was growing up, my dad's parents' house meant three things: playing for hours in the playhouse in their yard, trying on old prom dresses in the attic with my cousin, and Waldorf salad with every single dinner. Granny's version was a very simple mix of apples, mayo, and raisins, but it is a dish evocative of some of the fondest memories of my childhood. Now if I could just figure out how to make her angel food cake allergy-free. . . . **SERVES 6**

1. Place the chopped apples in a mixing bowl and toss them with the lemon juice. Add in the celery, grapes, and yogurt. Toss to coat.

2. Sprinkle the salad with the sunflower seeds and toss again.

3. Serve in compote cups. The leftover salad can be stored, refrigerated, up to a day in an airtight container.

Note: If you are able to find only unsalted sunflower seeds in your supermarket, stir ¼ teaspoon of salt into the coconut milk yogurt before adding.

1 pound sweet apples (such as Fuji), diced
2 teaspoons lemon juice
1 rib celery, sliced
⅓ cup quartered red grapes
¼ cup plain coconut milk yogurt
1 tablespoon roasted, salted sunflower seeds (optional)

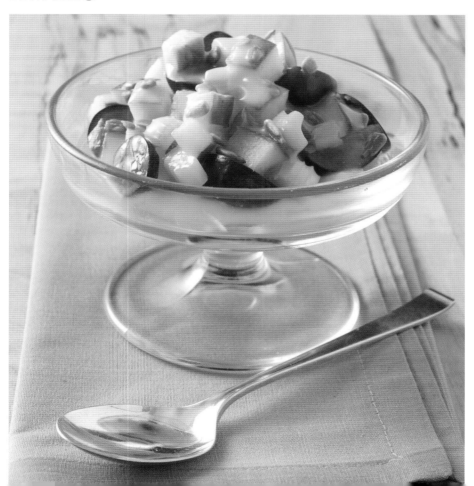

Tabbouleh

Last year I got to thinking about tabbouleh and how much I loved it before I was diagnosed with my food allergies. I associated many a happy memory with it, but I wasn't quite sure what I missed most about it. And then it hit me: color. I love colorful food. So I pondered how I could make a beautiful, fresh, and colorful version that wouldn't make me sick, and then it came to me: red quinoa complemented by green and red vegetables. My taste buds and food memories of yesteryear did not steer me wrong. I highly recommend this as a side dish for a weeknight dinner, or toss in some chicken breast for a complete meal. SERVES 4

2 cups Chicken Stock (page 112), vegetable stock, or water

1 cup red or white quinoa

1 cup chopped Italian parsley leaves (about 1 small bunch)

3 Roma tomatoes, seeded and diced

2 scallions, white and light green parts, chopped

1 medium cucumber, peeled, seeded, and diced

¼ cup mint, roughly torn

½ teaspoon minced garlic

1 tablespoon olive oil

¼ cup fresh-squeezed lemon juice

1. Put the stock or water and quinoa in a saucepan and bring to a boil. Reduce to a simmer, cover, and cook for about 15 minutes or until the liquid has been absorbed. Remove from the heat to cool.

2. In a large bowl combine the parsley, tomatoes, scallions, cucumber, mint, and garlic; set aside.

3. Make the dressing by whisking together the oil and lemon juice in a separate, small bowl.

4. Combine the vegetable and herb mixture with the cooled quinoa, and then pour the dressing over the top. Toss to combine.

4. Let the tabbouleh chill for at least an hour or even overnight before serving. Chilling for at least an hour allows all the flavors to fully absorb. Leftovers may be stored in an airtight container, refrigerated, for up to 3 days.

Note: Red quinoa is an heirloom variety of quinoa that is available in most supermarkets. If you are unable to find it, this recipe works just as well with white quinoa.

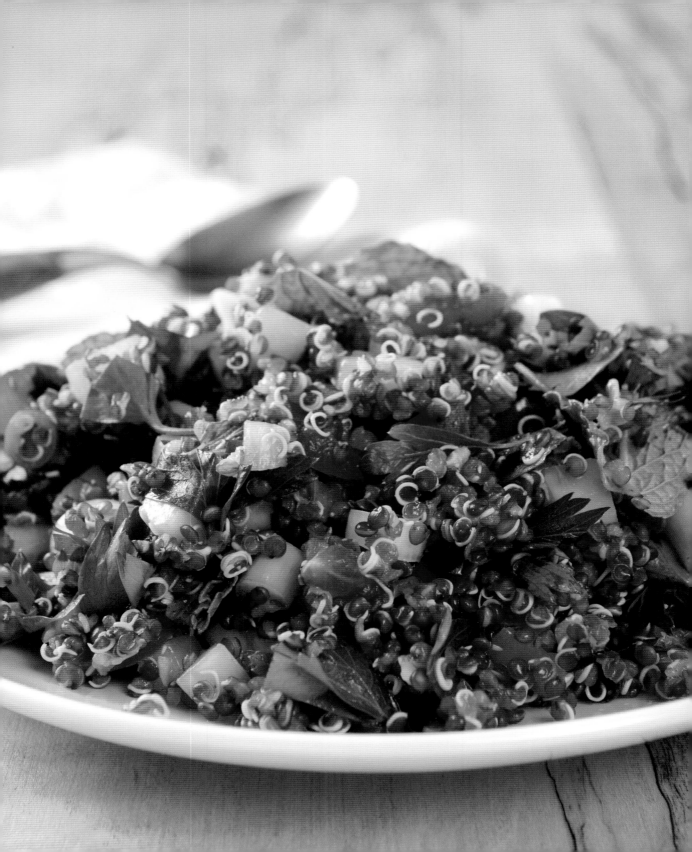

Shredded Carrot Salad

My mother fed this to us all the time as children, and I see it in delis all over New York City. There is just something about the combination of the plump, juicy, sweet raisins and the crisp, shredded carrots that makes my mouth water. I'm still a sucker for this salad that my mom used to fool us into eating our vegetables, and though I don't have to coax my girls into eating carrots because they already love them, I serve this as a healthy side with dinner all the time. SERVES 4

2 cups shredded carrots
¼ cup red raisins
3 tablespoons plain coconut milk yogurt
¾ teaspoon lemon juice
¼ teaspoon salt

1. Place the carrots and raisins in a large salad bowl.

2. In a small bowl whisk together the yogurt, lemon juice, and salt.

3. Pour the dressing over the carrots and raisins and toss to combine.

4. Leftovers may be stored, refrigerated, in an airtight container for up to 3 days, though this salad is best eaten on the day it is made.

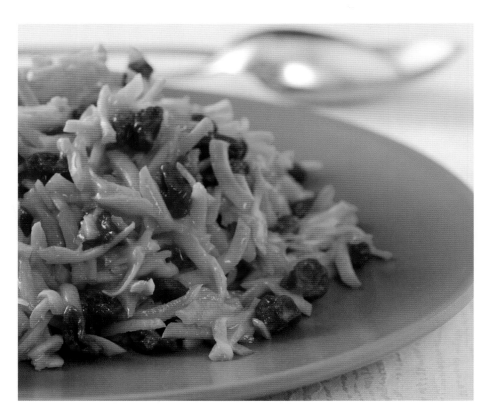

Corn Salad

I love corn salad. There is something about the combination of sweet, crisp corn, spicy peppers, and a twist of lime juice that gets me every time. Corn, fresh from the farm out on Long Island, is so sweet and crisp in mid-July that I love to make this at least once a week and keep it on hand as a side for lunch and dinner the whole week. If you prefer to make this year-round, frozen corn works just fine, too. **SERVES 6**

1. Steam the ears of corn just until the corn turns bright yellow and starts to smell of corn, about 5 to 7 minutes. Drain the water and rinse the ears of corn with cold water until they are cool to the touch. Cut the kernels from the cobs into a large salad bowl.

2. Add the diced red pepper, lime juice, cilantro, jalapeño, and salt. Toss the salad to combine all the ingredients.

3. You may serve this immediately, but I like to cover it and let the flavors marinate overnight before serving.

Note: The leftovers may be stored, refrigerated, up to 5 days in an airtight container.

6 ears corn, shucked, or 4 cups frozen corn

$1/2$ cup diced red bell pepper (about $1/2$ small pepper)

2 tablespoons lime juice (about the juice of 2 limes)

1 tablespoon finely chopped cilantro

1 level tablespoon finely chopped jalapeño, seeds and ribs removed to reduce the heat (about $1/2$ small jalapeño)

1 teaspoon salt

Pasta Salad

Have you ever been to a summer potluck that hasn't included a pasta salad? I haven't! This salad calls for a light vinaigrette instead of a heavy mayonnaise-based dressing, and it's a great way to sneak in lots of colorful, spring- and summertime vegetables. Because of the nature of rice pasta, I find that too much of the dressing gets absorbed to eat it the next day. This healthy salad is best mixed up, dressed, and eaten right away. Do not let my selection of vegetables limit you: Carrots, red pepper, and various fresh herbs work well in this salad, too. SERVES 8–10

1 pound rice pasta

1/3 cup frozen peas, thawed

3/4 cup diced zucchini (about 1/2 small)

3/4 cup asparagus tips (from about 20 spears)

20 cherry tomatoes, cut into thirds

1/4 cup freshly squeezed lemon juice

1/4 cup olive oil

1 clove garlic, pressed

1/2 teaspoon salt

1/2 teaspoon chopped fresh rosemary

1. Cook the pasta according to the package directions, adding the peas in the last 5 minutes; drain and rinse with cold water.

2. While the pasta is cooking, steam the zucchini and asparagus in another pot until they are crisp-tender, about 5 to 7 minutes.

3. While the vegetables are steaming, fill a large bowl with cold water and ice. When the zucchini and asparagus are steamed, use a slotted spoon to transfer them to the ice water to stop the cooking; drain. Toss together the pasta, peas, zucchini, asparagus, and cherry tomatoes.

4. Whisk together the lemon juice, olive oil, garlic, salt, and chopped rosemary in a small bowl. Dress the pasta salad just before serving; toss and serve.

5. The salad is best eaten right away, but the leftovers may be stored in an airtight container, refrigerated, for up to 3 days.

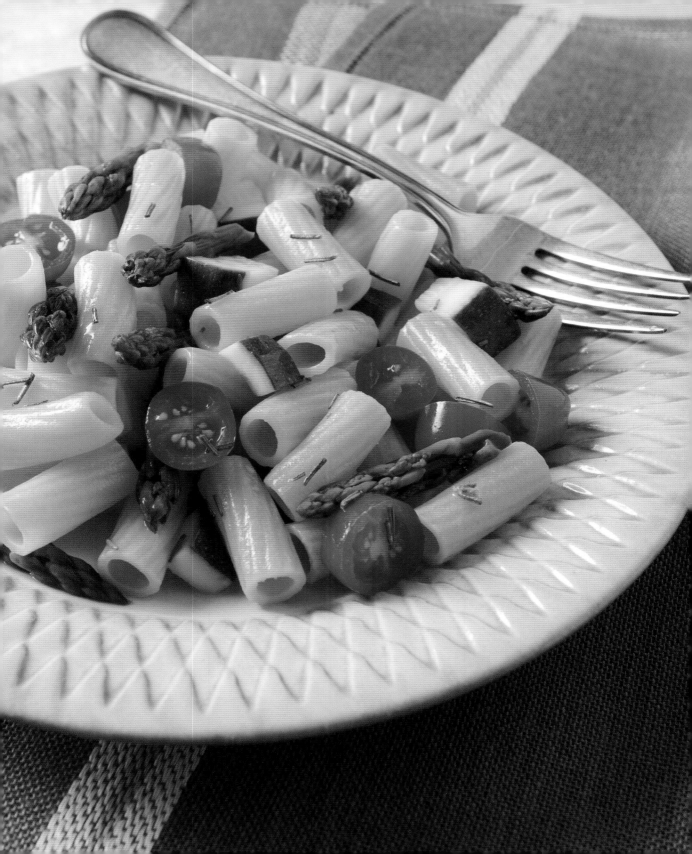

Cucumber Salad

This is one of my favorite salads to make, as it is evocative of my time studying in Germany as a college student. This was the German equivalent to American baked beans at barbecues, because it is so easy to make that everyone has a recipe for it. It is so refreshing, and since my children actually like cucumbers, it usually goes over really well. A true classic, it is not only the perfect picnic accompaniment, but also the perfect thing to make if you are short on time. Try mounding a little on a slice of my Crusty White Bread (page 136) spread with dairy- and soy-free margarine for a filling snack. SERVES 6

3 cucumbers, peeled (about 2 pounds)

¼ small red onion

1 teaspoon chopped fresh dill

½ teaspoon salt

Dash black pepper

3 tablespoons red wine vinegar

3 tablespoons canola oil

1. Slice the cucumbers thin on a mandoline set to ⅛ inch and place them in a large salad bowl.

2. Thinly, vertically sliver the onion and add it to the bowl. Sprinkle the cucumber and the onion with the dill.

3. In a small bowl, whisk together the salt, pepper, vinegar, and oil, and pour this vinaigrette over the cucumber and onions. Serve right away.

Note: This salad is best on the day that it is made, because the acidity of the vinegar makes the cucumbers soften. However, leftovers may be stored in an airtight container, refrigerated, overnight.

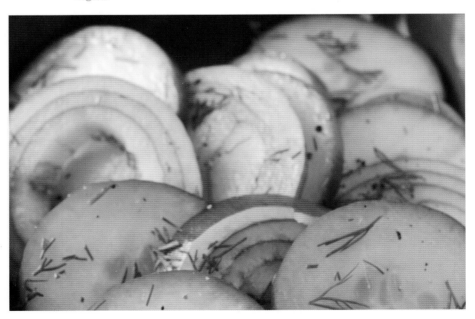

Charoset

When I married my husband, I had never been to a traditional Jewish celebration, so I was completely unfamiliar with the food. However, I found that I liked the sound of most of the dishes. Unfortunately most of the wheat-laden, eggy kugels and the matzoh do not agree with my immune system. What I immediately loved, though, was the charoset served at Passover. The Passover Seder is usually very long, and by the time that we get to this dish, I am starving! Here is a tasty, nut-free version for your Seder table or, really, any day of the year. SERVES 8

1. Combine all the ingredients in the bowl of a food processor. Pulse for a few seconds or until the mixture is a coarse dice. Serve.

2. Store leftovers in the refrigerator in an airtight container for 2 to 3 days.

2 cups peeled and cored sweet apples
1 cup yellow raisins
2 tablespoons red wine
1½ teaspoons honey
½ teaspoon cinnamon
¼ teaspoon ginger

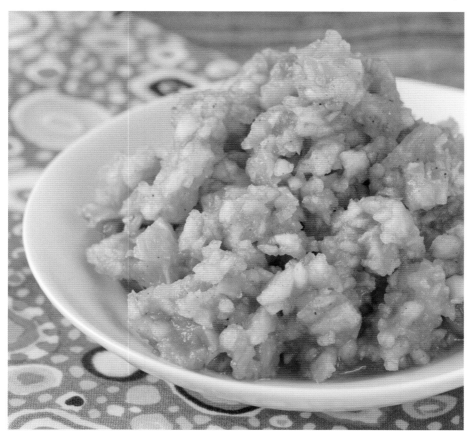

Coleslaw

Tangy yet sweet, full of fiber, and delicious atop my Shredded Pork Sandwiches (page 88), coleslaw is something that shows up everywhere in the summertime. A true family favorite, coleslaw tastes great with everything from a burger to a basket of hush puppies to barbecue. SERVES 6

2 pounds green cabbage,
  cored and shredded
1/2 cup shredded carrots
1 1/2 teaspoons salt
3 tablespoons sugar
1/2 teaspoon celery seed
3 tablespoons cider vinegar
3 tablespoons canola oil
Dash pepper

1. Place the shredded cabbage and carrots in a mesh colander and sprinkle with the salt. Toss to combine and then let stand to drain for 1 hour. Press to squeeze out the water and then transfer the carrots and cabbage to a large bowl.

2. In a small bowl, whisk together the sugar, celery seed, cider vinegar, canola oil, and pepper. Pour the dressing over the shredded vegetables and toss to combine.

3. Cover the bowl and let the flavors ripen for 2 hours before serving. This coleslaw is best eaten on the day it's made.

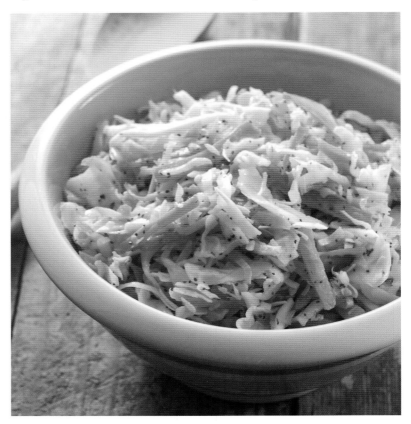

Tomato and Hominy Salad

I only discovered hominy, which is simply corn with the germ and hull removed, after I was diagnosed with food allergies, but I have to admit that I really love it. Hominy can be found, canned, in most local supermarkets. Popular in Southern cooking and in Latin American fare such as posole, hominy is delicious and unexpected when used in American cooking, and a great gluten-free alternative to pasta. I particularly like to serve this take on hominy as a side with chicken soft tacos. SERVES 4

1. Preheat the oven to 400°F and line a rimmed baking sheet with parchment paper. Place the tomatoes on the prepared baking sheet and roast for 20 minutes.

2. While the tomatoes are roasting, place the hominy, scallions, and cilantro in a large bowl. Sprinkle with the lime juice, salt, and pepper and toss to combine.

3. When the tomatoes come out of the oven, add them to the hominy mix and toss the salad again. Serve immediately.

Note: Leftovers may be stored in an airtight container, refrigerated, for up to 3 days.

1 pound grape tomatoes
2 15-ounce cans hominy, drained
3 scallions, chopped
1/4 cup chopped cilantro
1 tablespoon lime juice
1/4 teaspoon salt
1/8 teaspoon pepper

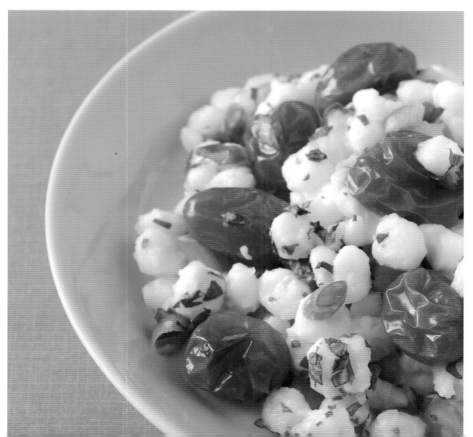

Traditional Dijon Vinaigrette

Green Goddess Vinaigrette

BBQ Sauce

Mayo

Egg-Free Caesar Salad Dressing

Ranch Dressing/Dip

Spicy Tomatillo Sauce

Croutons

All-Purpose Breading

All-Purpose Savory Pastry

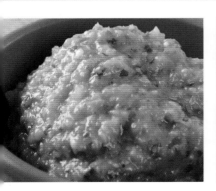
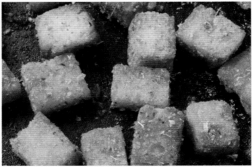
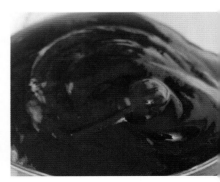

Condiments, Dressings, and Basics

Since being diagnosed with food allergies, I have given up most condiments. Because I am allergic to eggs, mayonnaise is no longer on my menu and creamy dressings like ranch and green goddess have also been stricken from my diet. Many bottled dressings and condiments contain modified food starch, making them unsafe for anyone avoiding wheat or gluten, and those that don't usually contain ingredients like high-fructose corn syrup, which I try to avoid unless I'm making candies. Enter this chapter. Tired of food that needed a little extra oomph, I wrote these recipes to give myself a little something to keep my sandwiches from being dry and to make my salads more piquant.

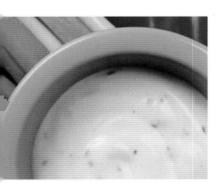
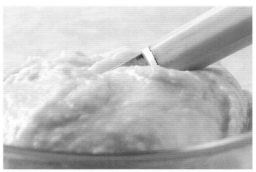
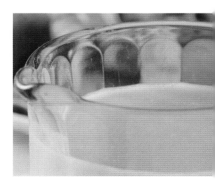

Traditional Dijon Vinaigrette

The versatility of this recipe is what makes it so special. I use this as a dressing for pasta salad, potato salad, or green salads, and it inevitably shows up at every single dinner party that we host. I especially love that I can switch lemon juice, sherry vinegar, or champagne vinegar for the red wine vinegar and end up with something completely new in flavor but equally as quick, simple, and reliable. MAKES ½ CUP

1 tablespoon good Dijon
　mustard (preferably Maille)
1 tablespoon red wine vinegar
Salt and pepper to taste
½ cup light extra-virgin
　olive oil

1. Combine the mustard, red wine vinegar, and salt and pepper in a bowl. Whisk in the olive oil in a steady stream until a thick emulsion forms. Serve immediately.

2. Store in an airtight container for up to a week. Bring to room temperature and whisk or shake well before serving.

Note: This dressing also may be made in the blender if it is easier for you to form the emulsion.

Green Goddess Vinaigrette

Before the advent of ranch dressing, green goddess was, perhaps, the most widely used salad dressing in America. The trouble with the traditional version is that it is made with both mayo and sour cream. So I decided to make this a light vinaigrette with all of the traditional flavors of the original. To make up for the lack of creaminess, I always serve this dressing with creamy avocado slices, shredded iceberg lettuce, and slivered red onions. MAKES ABOUT ½ CUP OF DRESSING, OR ENOUGH FOR A SALAD FOR 6

2 tablespoons minced fresh
　chervil
2 tablespoons minced fresh
　tarragon
2 tablespoons minced chives
1 teaspoon anchovy paste
　(optional)
¾ teaspoon salt
¼ cup lemon juice
½ cup light olive oil

1. Place the chervil, tarragon, and chives in the pitcher of a blender. Pulse to chop the herbs.

2. Add in the anchovy paste, if using, salt, and lemon juice and blend again, just to mix. With the blender on, pour in the oil in a slow, steady stream and continue blending until the vinaigrette emulsifies.

3. Pour the vinaigrette over a salad, toss, and serve immediately. The vinaigrette can be stored, covered, in the refrigerator for up to 1 day.

BBQ Sauce

When I lived down South, you absolutely could not go to a tailgate party or picnic without barbecue pork sandwiches being served. Barbecue stands are everywhere down there, and everyone is a barbecue connoisseur. I love barbecue and wanted to make a version that wasn't loaded with corn syrup and modified food starch like a lot of the commercial brands. I think that you will be overjoyed with the results. MAKES 2 CUPS

1. Combine all the ingredients in a large bowl until the sauce is smooth and all the ingredients are thoroughly incorporated.

2. Make this ahead and store it for up to 1 week in the refrigerator.

2 cups corn syrup-free ketchup
2 tablespoons vinegar
2 tablespoons plus 1 teaspoon brown sugar
2 tablespoons plus 1 teaspoon molasses
1 teaspoon dry mustard
¼ teaspoon celery seed
1 teaspoon salt
¾ teaspoon cumin
¼ teaspoon ground cayenne pepper
¼ teaspoon garlic salt
1 tablespoon lemon juice
½ teaspoon allspice

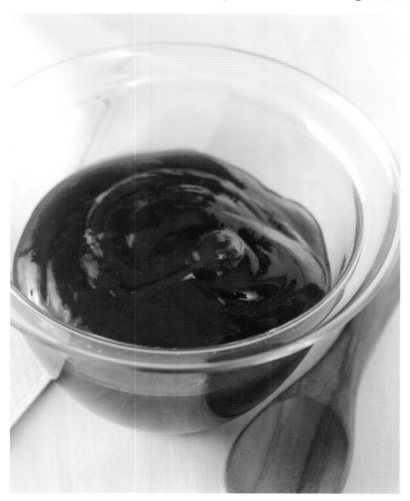

Mayo

I used to love sandwiches slathered with mayonnaise. However, my egg allergy keeps me from eating it. I attempted to make this in more traditional ways by creating an emulsion with an acid and oil, but it turned out more like a thin salad dressing. Then I attempted to make it from a nondairy milk thickened with xanthan gum. That was just slimy and gross. Finally, I was working on my rosemary and white bean hummus when it occurred to me that the white beans get so creamy and have such a neutral taste that I could season them like mayonnaise, and this is what I ended up with. It is delicious spread on my Crusty White Bread (see page 136) and then layered with bacon, lettuce, and tomato. MAKES ¾ CUP

1 19-ounce can cannellini beans, drained and 3 tablespoons liquid reserved
1 teaspoon lemon juice
1 teaspoon dry mustard
1 teaspoon white wine vinegar
½ teaspoon salt
¼ cup olive oil

1. Place the drained beans in the bowl of a food processor with the lemon juice, dry mustard, white wine vinegar, and salt. Process mixture until smooth, stop the motor, and then scrape down the sides of the bowl.

2. Turn on the food processor again and add the olive oil in a steady stream with the motor running; process for 1 minute.

3. Add in the reserved liquid and process again. Scrape down the sides once more. If the mayo is not completely smooth, process it for 1 more minute. Leftover mayo may be stored in an airtight container, refrigerated, for 3 to 5 days.

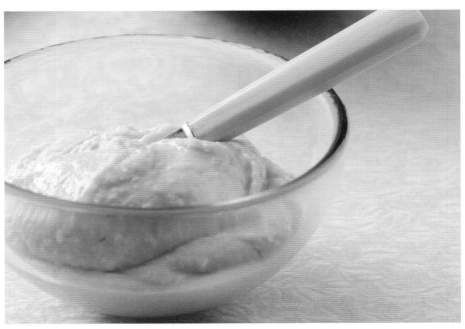

Egg-Free Caesar Salad Dressing

Oh, how I have missed Caesar salad! I love, love, love it, and now I can have it. I know that anchovy can be troublesome for some allergies, so feel free to omit it. The garlic really is the key to this recipe. This makes a lot of dressing, so reserve any leftovers for lunch the next day. MAKES 1¼ CUPS DRESSING, OR ENOUGH TO DRESS A VERY LARGE SALAD MADE FROM 2 LARGE HEADS OF ROMAINE LETTUCE, SHREDDED

1. Place the garlic cloves, Dijon mustard, salt, lemon juice, and anchovy paste, if using, in the pitcher of a blender. Blend on high until the mixture is thoroughly combined and the garlic is completely minced.

2. With the blender on high, slowly pour in the olive oil in a steady stream through the opening in the blender lid until a thick emulsion forms. Adjust the salt if necessary; serve immediately.

3. Store leftovers in an airtight container, refrigerated, up to 2 days. Shake very well before using the leftovers.

4 cloves garlic
2 tablespoons good Dijon mustard (preferably Maille)
¼ teaspoon salt
½ cup lemon juice
½ teaspoon anchovy paste (optional)
1 cup extra-virgin olive oil

Croutons

Oh yum! I just love croutons in a salad, and these go especially well with my Egg-Free Caesar Salad Dressing (see page 63) and some romaine lettuce. MAKES 2 CUPS

½ loaf Crusty White Bread (see page 136)

¼ cup olive oil

1 clove garlic

½ teaspoon dried parsley flakes

¼ teaspoon salt

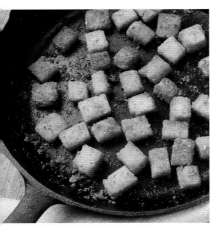

1. Preheat the oven to 425°F.

2. Cut off the crust of the bread and cut the remainder into cubes.

3. Blend the olive oil and garlic in a food processor until smooth. Stir in the dried parsley flakes and salt.

4. Pour the oil mixture into a large, ovenproof skillet and heat over medium heat. When the oil is hot, add the cubed bread and toss to coat. Cook the bread over medium heat, stirring constantly until the bread is thoroughly soaked in the oil and turning golden.

5. Place the entire pan in the preheated oven and bake the croutons for 12 minutes.

6. Remove the croutons from the oven, let them cool for 10 minutes, and use them immediately. The croutons will be warm and slightly crispy, and this is how I prefer to eat my croutons. However, for very hard croutons, leave them out overnight to get stale. The croutons are best eaten on the day they are made. Store any leftovers in an airtight container at room temperature overnight.

All-Purpose Breading

I love to bread things now that I can! Kids seem to be more inclined to eat breaded things, and this breading is so tasty and versatile that it works in lots of different recipes. Whether you fry this or bake it, it works well every time. Feel free to increase the amount of cayenne pepper if you love a little extra heat, or you can reduce it for finicky eaters. MAKES 2¾ CUPS

2 cups regular rice flour

½ cup cornmeal

2 tablespoons onion salt

2 tablespoons garlic powder

1 tablespoon paprika

1 teaspoon cayenne pepper

1. Whisk all of the ingredients together in a large mixing bowl.

2. Store the completed mix in an airtight container, refrigerated, for up to 3 months, using as needed.

All-Purpose Savory Pastry

As I was developing recipes for this book, I noticed that the pastries for my empanadas and pigs in a blanket were similar, and that the same pastry could easily be used as a pizza crust, too. As a Midwesterner, I prefer a thicker, chewier, Chicago-style pizza crust to a thin, crispy New York crust, and this recipe fits the bill. Given that it worked so well for everything from a wrapper for a cocktail frank to a savory hand pie, I decided to make one key pastry recipe. I use this pastry all the time, and I think that it will become a staple in your repertoire as well. MAKES 1 16-INCH PIZZA CRUST, 30 PIGS IN A BLANKET, OR 6 EMPANADAS

1. In a large glass measuring cup, sprinkle the yeast over the warm water and stir in the sugar. Let stand to proof for 10 minutes. It should be very foamy after 10 minutes.

2. While the yeast is proofing, add the Chinese rice flour, potato starch, sorghum flour, baking soda, baking powder, salt, and xanthan gum to a large bowl and whisk together well.

3. In the bowl of a stand mixer, cream together the organic palm fruit oil shortening and applesauce. Pour the cider vinegar into the liquid ingredients and in three alternating additions, add the dry and wet ingredients, mixing well after each addition.

4. Gather the dough into a ball with well-floured hands (I use additional sorghum flour) and then use the dough according to the recipe directions.

Note: When I make this, I prefer to roll it out on a very well-floured surface with a well-floured rolling pin, using sorghum flour for dusting. However, my mother insists that the only way to roll this out is on a well-floured pastry cloth.

1 package rapid-rise yeast
1$^{1}/_{4}$ cups warm water (105°F)
1 tablespoon granulated sugar
2$^{1}/_{2}$ cups Chinese rice flour
$^{3}/_{4}$ cup potato starch
$^{1}/_{2}$ cup sorghum flour
1 teaspoon baking soda
1 teaspoon baking powder
1 teaspoon salt
2 teaspoons xanthan gum
$^{1}/_{4}$ cup organic palm fruit oil shortening
$^{1}/_{4}$ cup plus 2 tablespoons unsweetened applesauce
1 tablespoon cider vinegar

Corn Dogs

Pot Roast

Shepherd's Pie

Marinated Flank Steak

Irish Stew

Brisket

Pan Gravy

Roast Beef

Tamale Pie

Pork Souvlaki

Sloppy Joe

Shredded Pork Sandwiches

Empanadas

Corned Beef and Cabbage

Stuffed Peppers

Weeknight Turkey Chili

Chicken Curry

Turkey Meat Loaf

Chicken Salad

Individual Chicken Potpies

Turkey, Red Pepper, Arugula,
and Hominy Soup

Lemon Rosemary Chicken Breasts

Chicken Soft Tacos

Fried Chicken

Perfect Roast Chicken

Chicken Stock

Turkey Meatballs

Pizza

Pupusas

Spring Risotto

Marinara Sauce

Black Beans and Yellow Rice

Black Bean Burgers

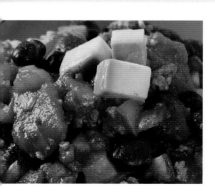
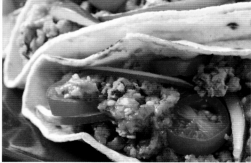
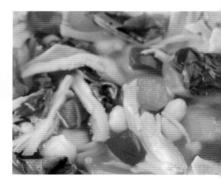

Main Courses

When I was growing up in Ohio, my parents bought a cow, a pig, and a lamb at the local fair every year and had them butchered for our annual meat supply. This way, we knew where our meat was coming from and that it had been raised in a responsible way. Living in New York City, without room for a deep freezer and no idea where to find a meat locker, we have, unfortunately, not been able to carry on this family tradition. However, I do buy organic meat as often as possible and usually buy from our butcher rather than at a regular supermarket so that I know what I am serving is fresh.

Chicken and turkey are also staples in my family's diet: chicken salad, chicken noodle soup, and chicken potpie are a few of our favorites. Like many dishes made with meat, the conventional versions of these recipes call for ingredients I can't eat. The recipe that spawned the idea for this entire book was the one I developed for chicken potpie. One day I was reminded of my childhood love of frozen potpie and really got a hankering for it. This craving led to the notion of a book about comfort foods. Once I had that recipe the floodgates opened, and all my old favorites like fried chicken and buffalo wings came to me.

Recently I have made an effort to feed my family more vegetarian fare. I had always had the idea that to be vegetarian, a meal must contain kelp and taste like cardboard. However, as I began experimenting with vegetarian cooking, I came to understand that meatless meals can be interesting and flavorful. Risotto and pizza are just two examples. In the summer, heavily laden with fresh vegetables, garlic, and herbs, pizza might be the most outstanding vegetarian comfort food of all.

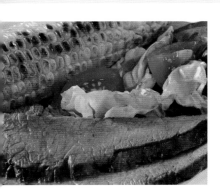 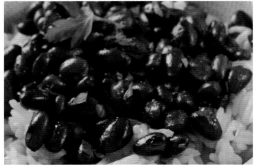 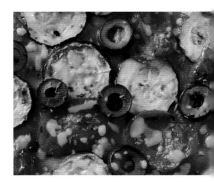

Corn Dogs

When I was a child, cornbread was one of my least favorite foods, because I had only ever tasted it at the school cafeteria. It wasn't something routinely served at home. But then I headed south and discovered that cornbread is one of life's great pleasures. So when I tasted my first corn dog, I could think of nothing better. A hot dog wrapped in cornbread? Totally, ridiculously delicious. I like to use Applegate Farms jumbo hot dogs for this recipe, because they are uncured and do not contain any soy, casein, or gluten. My oldest daughter has been asking to go to Coney Island for her birthday, so I'm thinking of serving these for the Coney Island–themed birthday dinner that we'll have afterward. SERVES 10

Canola oil for frying
1 recipe Hush Puppies batter
    (see page 126)
10 ice pop sticks
10 all-beef, uncured, soy-free
    hot dogs

1. Fill a fryer with the canola oil according to the fryer directions or fill a large skillet with 3 to 4 inches of canola oil. Preheat the fryer or the oil in the skillet to 350°F.

2. Prepare the hush puppies batter according to the recipe directions.

3. Push one ice pop stick about a third of the way into each hot dog. Scoop out 1 tablespoon of the hush puppies batter and, using your fingers, press the first scoop of batter around the bottom third of the hot dog. Scoop another 1 tablespoon of batter and press it around the middle of the hot dog, and then repeat one more time, covering the top of the hot dog.

4. Fry the corn dogs, one at a time so as not to overcrowd the fryer, for about 3 minutes or until they are completely golden brown. If a corn dog sticks to the bottom of the fryer basket, gently remove it with tongs, so as not to dislodge the corn coating.

5. Remove the cooked corn dogs to a paper towel–lined plate to drain.

6. These corn dogs taste best served immediately, but completely cooled corn dogs may be frozen in an airtight container for up to 3 months and reheated in a 450°F oven for 15 minutes.

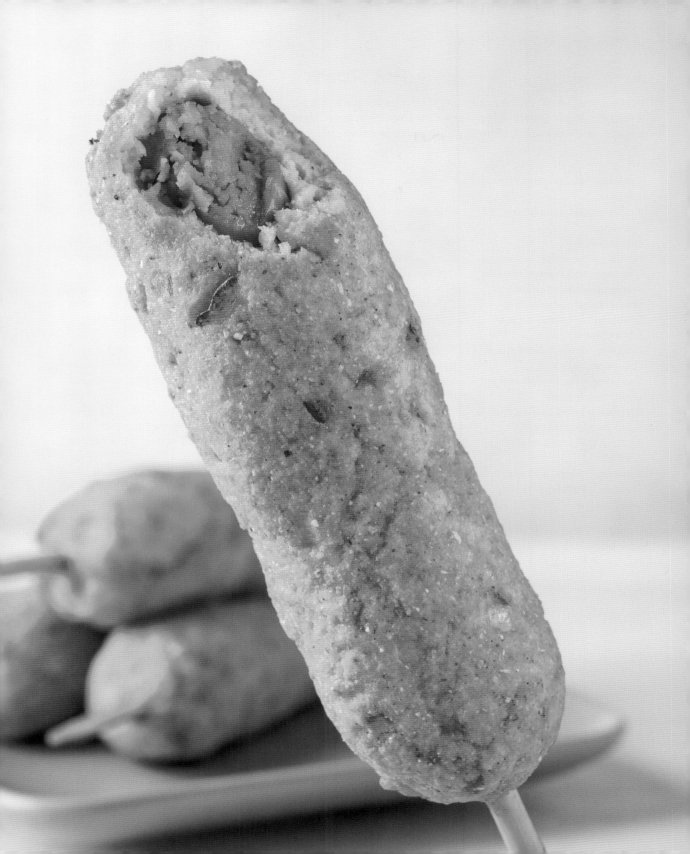

Pot Roast

When all else fails, make pot roast! Throw everything in a pot, cook for a few hours, and out comes a nutritious dinner that takes very little hands-on time. My mother used to make this at least once a week, and I serve it frequently in the winter when I want to have a cozy, but easy dinner. SERVES 8

3 pounds boneless beef chuck roast

2 tablespoons canola oil, divided

1 teaspoon salt

1 large yellow onion, cut into 8 wedges and then broken up

1 tablespoon fresh thyme

1 tablespoon cornstarch

2 tablespoons tomato paste

1 cup red wine

2 cups gluten-free beef stock

1 bay leaf

3 large carrots, peeled and cut into 1-inch coins

2 large parsnips, peeled and cut into 1-inch coins

3 celery stalks, cut into 1-inch slices

2 pounds Yukon Gold potatoes, scrubbed and quartered

1. Preheat the oven to 350°F.

2. Rub the roast with 1 tablespoon of the canola oil and the salt. In a large pot with a tightly fitting lid or a Dutch oven, heat the remaining tablespoon of canola oil over medium-high heat. Add the roast and brown all four sides for 2 minutes per side. Remove the pot from the heat and remove the roast to a plate.

3. Add the onions to the pot. Sprinkle the onions with the thyme and cornstarch. Coat the onion mixture with the tomato paste.

4. Return the roast to the pot, placing it atop the onions. Pour in the wine and beef stock and add the bay leaf. Firmly place the lid on top of the pot. Place the pot or Dutch oven in the oven and bake for 1½ hours.

5. Remove the roast from the oven and add the carrots, parsnips, celery, and potatoes. Return to the oven and roast for an additional hour.

6. Remove the roast from the oven and slice. Serve with the vegetables and potatoes and drizzle with the juices from the bottom of the pan. Store leftovers in an airtight container, refrigerated, for up to 3 days.

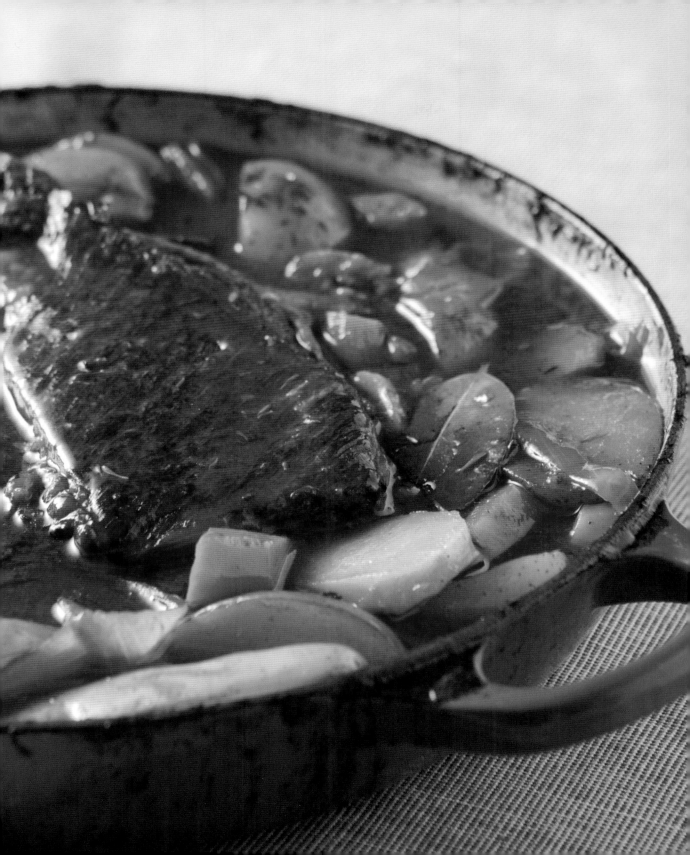

Shepherd's Pie

I often find myself with lots of leftovers at the end of the week: vegetables, mashed potatoes, and ground meat. Here's the perfect thing to use them up. If you don't like lamb, feel free to substitute ground beef or ground turkey. SERVES 8

1 recipe Rosemary Smashed
    Potatoes (see page 128)
2 teaspoons olive oil
¼ cup diced yellow onions
1 cup diced carrots (about 2
    medium carrots)
1 pound ground lamb
1 teaspoon salt
¼ teaspoon pepper
3 tablespoons tomato paste
¼ cup water
½ cup frozen peas, thawed

1. Prepare the Rosemary Smashed Potatoes according to the recipe directions. Then preheat the oven to 400°F.

2. Heat the oil in a large skillet and sauté the onions until they are soft and translucent, about 3 minutes. Add the carrots and continue cooking until they soften, about 7 to 8 minutes. Add the lamb, breaking it up with a wooden spoon as it cooks. Cook the lamb until it is cooked through and then drain off the excess fat. Add the salt, pepper, tomato paste, and water. Stir the lamb mixture until it is completely coated with tomato paste. Stir in the peas.

3. Spoon the lamb mixture into a 9-inch deep-dish pie plate and cover it with the Rosemary Smashed Potatoes. Smooth out the potatoes with a fork to create a decorative pattern on the potatoes, pushing them all the way to the edge of the pie plate.

4. Bake the pie in the preheated oven for 10 to 15 minutes or until the potatoes begin to pull away from the sides of the pan and are just golden at the edge. Serve immediately.

5. Leftovers may be stored in an airtight container, refrigerated, for up to 3 days.

Note: The constructed, fully cooled but unbaked pie may also be tightly covered and frozen for up to 3 months. Remove from the freezer when you are ready to use it, and bake in a 400°F oven for 55 to 60 minutes.

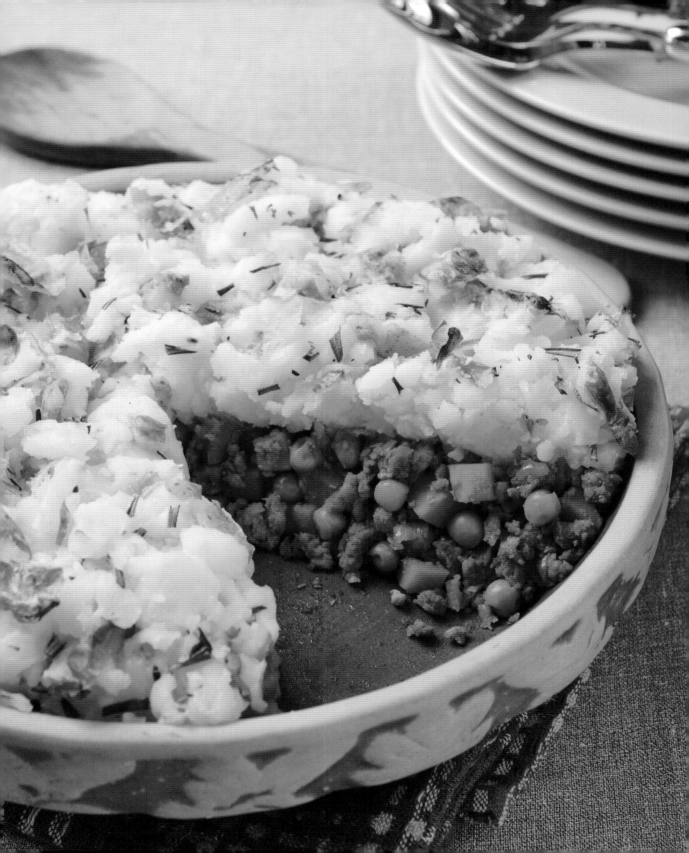

Marinated Flank Steak

We entertain a lot on the weekends in the summer, but I hate cleaning up. So this is my go-to main course. I can marinate it the day before and grill it while I wash the pan. All this needs is a salad and some corn on the cob to make it a complete meal. SERVES 6-8

¼ cup balsamic vinegar
½ cup olive oil
1 teaspoon salt
2 cloves garlic, minced
Dash black pepper
1¾ pounds flank steak

1. In a small bowl whisk together the vinegar, oil, salt, garlic, and pepper.

2. Place the steak in a nonreactive pan or in a large ziplock bag. Pour the marinade over the steak, cover the pan with plastic wrap or seal the bag, and marinate in the refrigerator for up to 24 hours.

3. Preheat the grill to high. Remove the meat from the marinade and place the steak on the preheated grill. Grill the steak 5 to 7 minutes per side for medium-rare steak.

4. Remove the steak to a platter and loosely tent it with aluminum foil. Allow the steak to rest for 10 minutes before slicing against the grain and serving.

5. Leftovers may be stored, refrigerated and covered, for up to 3 days.

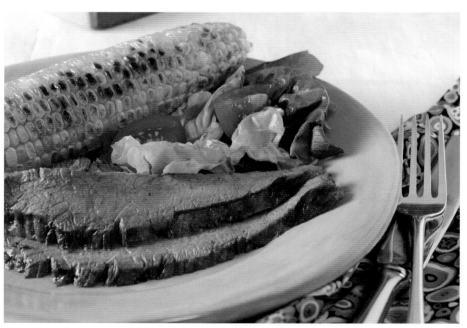

Irish Stew

My mother made stew at least once a week when I was growing up, and for as much as I complained about it at the time, I secretly loved it and still do. No matter what, this stew makes the house smell wonderful on a winter day, and since I make it far less than once a week, I never get a complaint when it comes to the table. **SERVES 6 GENEROUSLY**

1. Preheat the oven to 350°F degrees.

2. Place the beef chuck in a large Dutch oven and toss it with the cornstarch to coat.

3. Add the tomato paste, new potatoes, onions, carrots, garlic, salt, sugar, bay leaves, thyme, balsamic vinegar, tomato puree, beef stock, and beer to the pot and stir just to combine. Place mixture, uncovered, over medium-high heat and bring to a boil. Remove the Dutch oven from the heat, cover it, and place it in the pre-heated oven.

4. Bake the stew for 2 hours and 15 minutes or until the beef is fork-tender and the sauce has thickened. Remove the stew from the oven and stir in the thawed peas.

5. Serve the stew immediately with my Crusty White Bread (page 136) or store the cooled stew in an airtight container for up to 5 days in the refrigerator. The completely cooled stew may also be frozen in an airtight container for up to 3 months.

2 pounds cubed beef chuck
1 tablespoon cornstarch
1 6-ounce can tomato paste
1 pound new potatoes, scrubbed and halved
1 large yellow onion, cut into wedges and broken up
2 large carrots, sliced
4 cloves garlic, slivered
1 teaspoon salt
1 tablespoon sugar
2 bay leaves
1 teaspoon dry thyme
1 tablespoon balsamic vinegar
$^3/_4$ cup canned tomato puree
2 $^3/_4$ cups gluten-free beef stock
$^3/_4$ cup gluten-free sorghum beer (see Where to Shop)
1 10-ounce package frozen peas, thawed

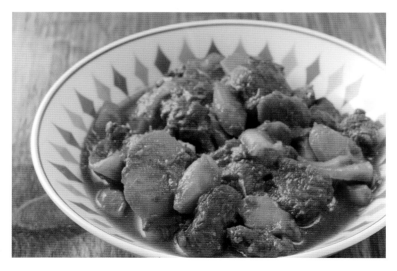

Brisket

It took a long time for me to come up with a good brisket recipe: I sat down with many brisket experts and talked it out. I went to the butcher for his two cents. I asked every Jewish grandma that I knew. Nothing worked. Then I asked my friend Lori if she had any suggestions, and I hit the brisket jackpot: The key to good brisket is patience. In order for the brisket to get tender, it must be cooked on very low heat for a very long time. Serve this brisket with my pan gravy (below) to make an extra-special dinner. **SERVES 8 GENEROUSLY**

1 2½-pound flat beef brisket
2 stalks celery, diced
1 large carrot, sliced
1 large yellow onion, cut in
    wedges and then broken up
1 teaspoon paprika
1 teaspoon chili powder
2 bay leaves
1 teaspoon salt
¼ cup tomato paste
2 cups Italian red table wine
3 cups gluten-free beef stock

1. Preheat the oven to 300°F.

2. Place the brisket in a large Dutch oven. Arrange the vegetables around the meat. Add the spices, bay leaves, and salt. Spoon in the tomato paste, wine, and stock. The liquids should almost cover the brisket, leaving only about 2 inches out of the liquid. Bring the mixture just to a boil over medium-high heat. Remove the Dutch oven from the heat and cover it.

3. Place the Dutch oven in the preheated oven and bake for 3 hours or until the brisket is fork-tender and nearly falls apart when poked with a fork.

4. Remove the Dutch oven from the oven and thinly slice the brisket against the grain. Serve the brisket with the vegetables and pan gravy (below) if desired.

5. Store leftovers in an airtight container, refrigerated, for up to 3 days.

Pan Gravy

1 cup pan juices from a
    cooked beef brisket
¼ cup cold water
2 tablespoons cornstarch
¼ teaspoon salt

1. Place the pan juices in a small saucepan.

2. In a small cup, mix the water and cornstarch, whisking the mixture until it is completely smooth.

3. Whisk the slurry into the pan juices and bring the gravy to a simmer. Simmer, whisking constantly for 1 minute, then stir in the salt. The gravy may be used immediately or stored for 3 days in the refrigerator in an airtight container.

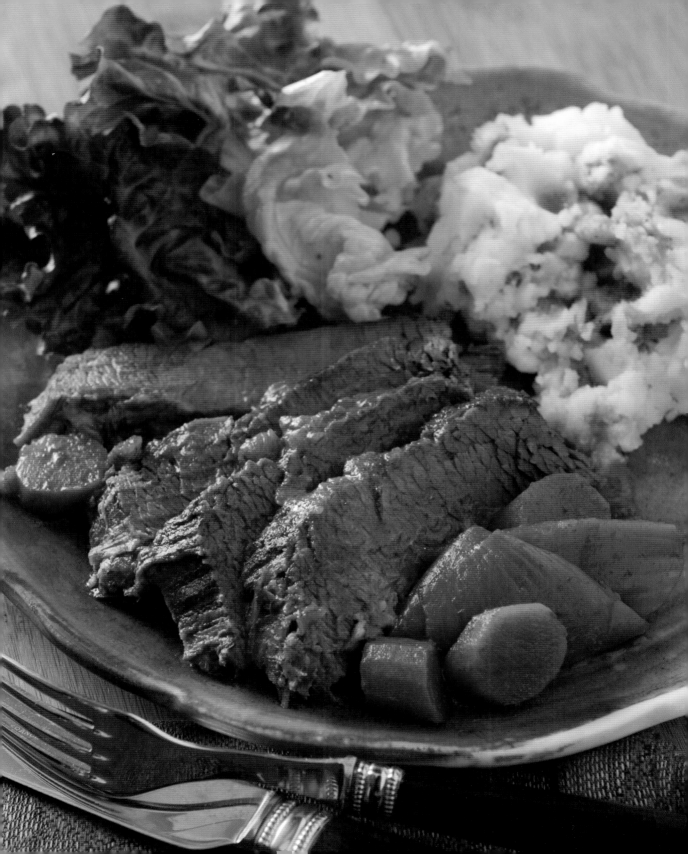

Roast Beef

Now that I have a white bread recipe (page 136) and a brown bread recipe (see page 130), I really love sandwiches again. Although the deli varieties are tasty, they often contain fillers such as corn syrup and soy, so I try not to eat them too often. I have found, though, that nothing beats homemade roast beef on sandwiches. Slice this recipe thin and serve it on my Crusty White Bread—make it au jus by reserving the pan juices for dipping, or slather with Dijon mustard. Either way, this is heavenly rare roast beef. SERVES 16

1 teaspoon salt
½ teaspoon black pepper
1 3-pound chuck roast
2 tablespoons olive oil
12 cloves garlic, peeled and
   sliced in half

1. Preheat the oven to 500°F.

2. Mix together the salt and pepper in a small bowl. Brush the roast with olive oil and rub it with the salt and pepper mixture so that it is evenly seasoned.

3. Make tiny slits in twenty-four places over the roast and shove the garlic cloves into the slits. Place the roast on a grate placed in the center of a roasting pan and put it in the preheated oven.

4. Bake the roast at 500°F for 24 minutes. Then turn off the heat. *Do not open the oven door.* Let the roast sit in the closed, unheated oven for 2 hours. After 2 hours, remove from the oven and slice thin.

5. Serve the sliced roast beef immediately, or you can store it, refrigerated, in an airtight container for up to 3 days.

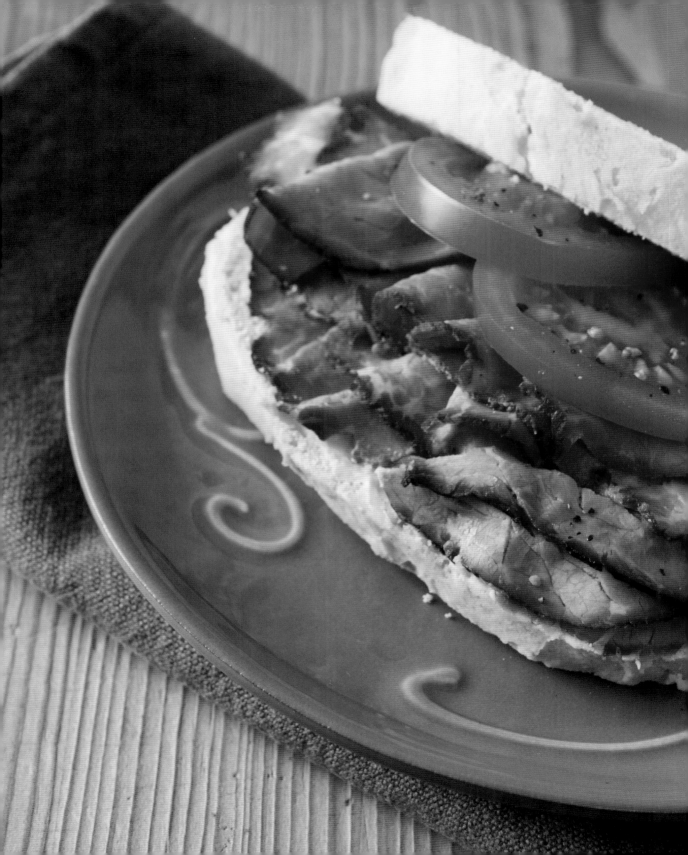

Tamale Pie

My grandmother sure loved to make casseroles, and this one is similar to one of her favorites. She did not cook often, but some of her Depression-era recipes stand out in my memory, because I think that those kinds of recipes inspired so many of today's classic comfort foods. During the Depression people had little money, so they had to take inexpensive ingredients and not only make them tasty and filling, but use every last scrap of leftover food. Hence, casseroles were popular because they left nothing to waste, and my tamale pie is a perfect example of frugal yet delicious cooking. Whenever I make tamale pie, I think of Granny and how happy she would be that my family has embraced casseroles, too. SERVES 8–10

4 1/2 cups water

1 teaspoon salt, divided

1 1/2 cups quick-cooking polenta

3/4 pound ground beef or ground turkey

1/2 teaspoon cumin

1/4 teaspoon chipotle powder

1 15-ounce can kidney beans, rinsed and drained

1 16-ounce jar mild salsa

1 cup Daiya cheese or appropriate cheese of your choice (optional)

1. Preheat the oven to 350°F.

2. Bring the water and 1/2 teaspoon salt to a boil in a large saucepan. When the water is boiling, slowly stir in the polenta with a large wooden spoon, stirring constantly to prevent clumping. When all the polenta has been stirred in and is smooth, turn the heat to low and cook for 5 minutes. Remove the polenta from the heat and scoop half of it into the bottom of a 9-inch deep-dish pie plate, spreading it evenly with a knife.

3. Brown the ground beef or turkey over medium-high heat in a large skillet, breaking up the meat as it cooks. Stir in the cumin, chipotle powder, and the remaining salt. When the meat is cooked through, remove it from the heat and pour off the excess fat. Return the meat to the burner.

4. Over medium heat, stir in the drained kidney beans and salsa. Cook the mixture just until the edges bubble.

5. Pour the meat mixture into the pie plate on top of the polenta. Spread the remaining polenta on top of the meat, making sure to spread it all the way to the edges of the pie plate.

6. Place the pie in the oven for 20 minutes. Remove from the oven, sprinkle with the cheese if using, and return to the oven for another 5 minutes.

7. Remove the pie from the oven and let it cool for 10 to 15 minutes before serving.

8. Store leftovers, covered and refrigerated, for up to 3 days.

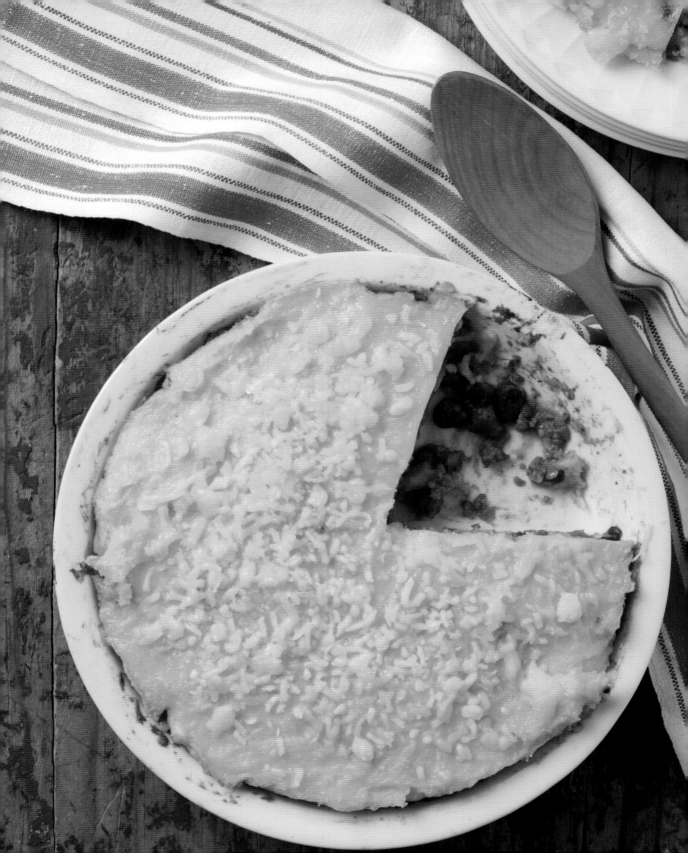

Pork Souvlaki

Whenever we go to our favorite Greek diner, this is what I get, without the pita, of course. Juicy and flavorful, my pork souvlaki is delicious and easy to make at home. Bake it or grill it for twenty minutes, but either way, it takes little prep time and always tastes great over rice with my dolmades (see page 30) as an appetizer or side. This version is lower in fat than what I get at the diner since it calls for pork tenderloin. SERVES 4

1½ pounds pork tenderloin
¼ cup olive oil
¼ cup lemon juice
1 tablespoon dried oregano
3 cloves garlic, minced
¼ teaspoon salt
⅛ teaspoon pepper
Tomato wedges and rice for
   serving

1. Place the pork tenderloin in a glass or ceramic, but not metal, rectangular baking dish. In a large bowl whisk together the olive oil, lemon juice, dried oregano, garlic, salt, and pepper. Pour this marinade over the pork tenderloin. Cover the pan with plastic wrap and refrigerate the pork for an hour.

2. After an hour turn over the pork so that it marinates evenly and return the covered pan to the refrigerator to marinate for another hour.

3. Preheat the oven to 400°F. Remove the plastic wrap from the pork tenderloin and pour off the marinade. Place the baking pan in the oven and roast the pork tenderloin for 20 to 25 minutes or until the internal temperature reads 160°F with an instant-read meat thermometer.

4. When the roast is finished, remove it from the oven and let it rest for 10 minutes. Cut the roast into cubes and serve over white rice with tomato wedges.

5. Leftovers may be stored in an airtight container, refrigerated, for up to 3 days.

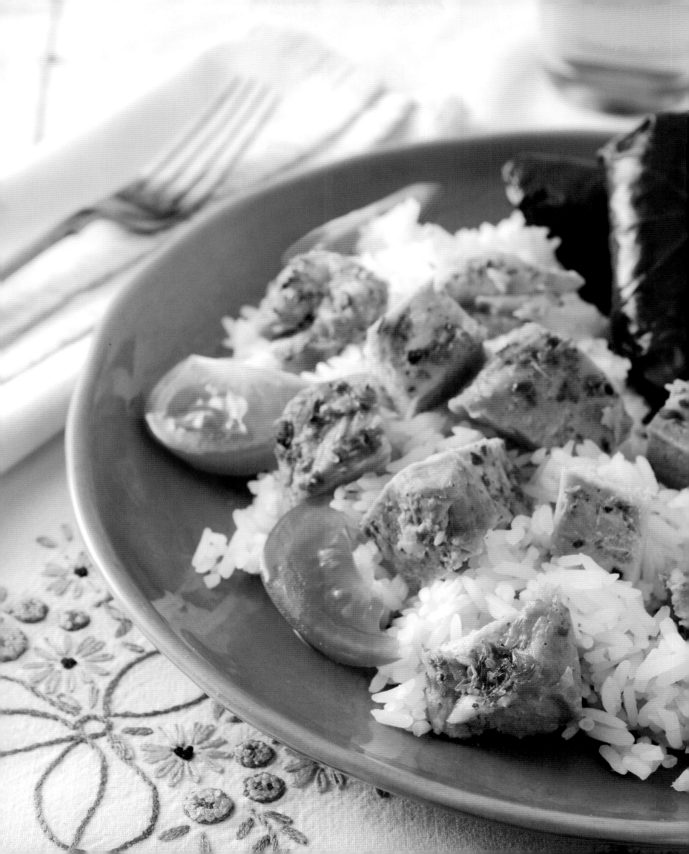

Sloppy Joe

Remember sloppy joe, the kind that came in a can, the kind filled with flour for thickening and corn syrup for, well, added flavor, I guess? Well, these are better. Gluten, dairy, soy, nut, and egg free, my sloppy joe takes about as long to make as that canned stuff takes to reheat, and it is equally delicious. My husband doesn't even like green peppers, and he gobbled this right up. After I took leftovers to my upstairs neighbors, they actually came and asked for more. These are sure to become a regular in your dinner repertoire. SERVES 6

1 pound ground sirloin

¼ cup diced onion (about 1 small)

½ small green bell pepper, diced

¾ cup corn syrup–free ketchup

1½ teaspoons dry mustard

1 tablespoon red wine vinegar

1 tablespoon brown sugar

3 tablespoons tomato paste

½ teaspoon garlic salt

½ teaspoon salt

¼ teaspoon black pepper

6 gluten-, dairy-, soy-, nut-, and egg-free hamburger buns (see Where to Shop)

1. Brown the ground sirloin in a large skillet over medium-high heat, breaking it up with a wooden spoon as it cooks. With a slotted spoon transfer the completely cooked meat to a plate. Tent the cooked sirloin with aluminum foil to keep the meat warm.

2. Meanwhile, in the same skillet, cook the onions and green peppers in the leftover fat until they are soft and the onions are translucent, about 5 to 7 minutes.

3. While the onions and green peppers are cooking, whisk together the ketchup, dry mustard, red wine vinegar, brown sugar, tomato paste, garlic salt, salt, and black pepper in a large bowl. Pour this sauce over the onions and green peppers and fold in the cooked meat. Cook over medium heat just until the sauce is warmed through.

4. Spoon ½ cup of the meat mixture onto the bottom half of each hamburger bun and serve immediately so that the buns do not get soggy.

5. Any leftover meat may be stored in an airtight container, refrigerated, for up to 3 days.

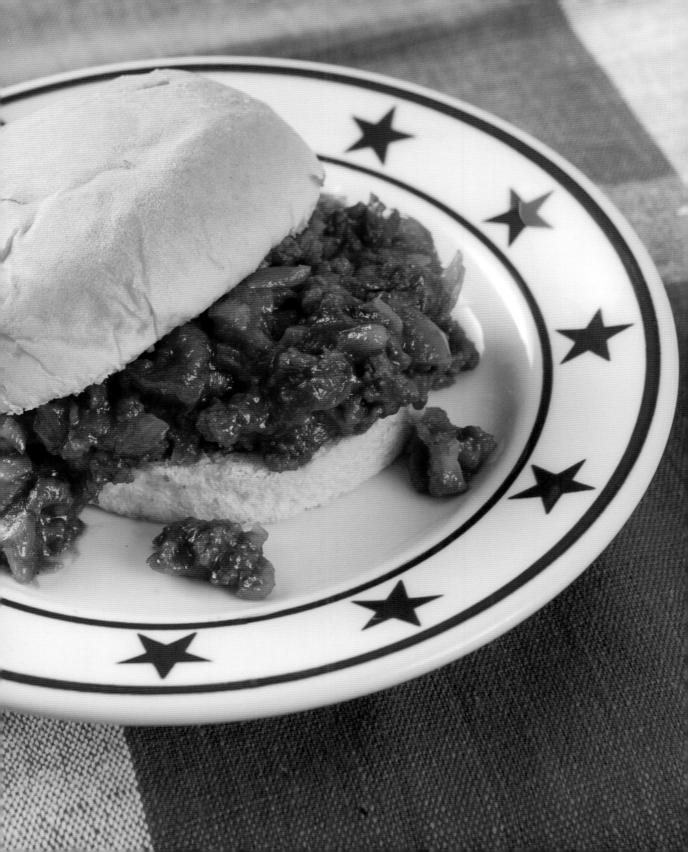

Shredded Pork Sandwiches

As I said in my description of my barbecue sauce (see page 61), shredded pork is a Southern institution. Barbecue restaurants are on every corner, the way that bagel stores abound in New York City. It was important to me that this shredded pork taste just the way I remember it tasting when I lived below the Mason-Dixon Line. Moist and tender, tangy and saucy, this shredded pork will surely become your new go-to when you are feeding a crowd. SERVES 12

5 pounds bone-in pork
   shoulder
1 tablespoon canola oil
1 teaspoon salt
¹⁄₈ teaspoon pepper
³⁄₄ cup water
1 ¹⁄₂ cups BBQ Sauce
   (see page 61)
12 gluten-, dairy-, soy-, nut-,
   and egg-free hamburger
   buns (see Where to Shop)

1. Preheat the oven to 325°F.

2. Remove the skin and all but about ¹⁄₄ inch of any remaining fat from the pork shoulder. Brush the roast with the canola oil. Mix together the salt and pepper and rub it into the pork roast. Place the roast, fat side up, in a large Dutch oven or large ovenproof pot fitted with a lid. Pour in the water and place the lid on top. Place the Dutch oven or pot in the preheated oven and roast the pork for 3 hours.

3. After 3 hours, check the roast. It should be very tender and falling apart, and an instant-read thermometer inserted in the roast should read 170°F.

4. Remove the Dutch oven or pot from the oven, remove the roast from the Dutch oven or pot, and let it rest for 10 minutes before shredding it with two forks. Discard the bone and any pieces of gristle or large pieces of fat.

5. When the pork is shredded, fold in the BBQ Sauce. Spoon about ¹⁄₂ cup of the shredded pork onto each bun and serve.

6. Serve the sandwiches immediately so that they don't get soggy. Leftover shredded pork may be stored in an airtight container, refrigerated, for up to 3 days.

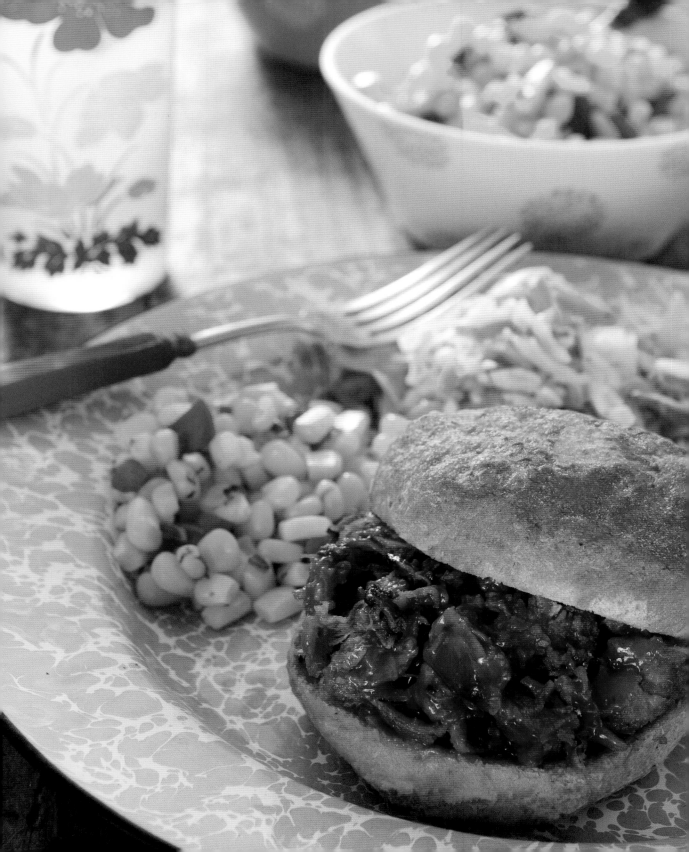

Empanadas

I actually pack my husband's lunch most days, so I am always trying to think of interesting things to send with him. I love to send a hand pie, or empanada, because he can pop it in the microwave to reheat it and eat it at his desk while he works. Sometimes it's nice to be able to forego protocol and just eat with your hands, especially when you are multitasking. When I make these for dinner, my kids love that they don't have to use utensils, and I love that I am getting some protein into them. We eat these at least once a week. Add a vegetable and you have a simple, quick, complete meal. MAKES 10–12 EMPANADAS

1 recipe All-Purpose Savory
   Pastry (see page 67)
2 teaspoons olive oil
1/4 cup diced onions (about 1
   small)
1/2 pound ground sirloin
1/4 teaspoon cumin
1/2 teaspoon salt
1/8 teaspoon pepper
1/4 cup sliced black olives
2 tablespoons tomato paste
2 tablespoons water
2 tablespoons yellow raisins

1. Preheat the oven to 375°F. Make the pastry according to the recipe directions.

2. Heat the olive oil in a large skillet over medium-high heat. Add the diced onions and sauté until soft and translucent, about 3 minutes. Add the sirloin and cook, breaking it up with a wooden spoon, until it is no longer pink. Remove the skillet from the heat and drain off any fat. Stir in the cumin, salt, pepper, black olives, tomato paste, water, and yellow raisins; set aside.

3. With a well-floured rolling pin on a well-floured surface (I use sorghum flour), roll out the pastry dough into an 18 x 24-inch rectangle. Cut the dough with a lightly greased 6-inch circular cutter.

4. Place 1 to 2 tablespoons of meat filling on half of the pastry circle and then fold it over. Press the edges together with a fork to seal the empanada. Place the finished empanadas on an ungreased baking sheet and bake in the preheated oven for 15 minutes.

5. Serve the empanadas immediately. Leftovers may be stored in an airtight container, refrigerated, for up to 3 days, or completely cooled empanadas may be frozen in an airtight container for up to 3 months.

Note: When I make these, I use the lightly greased rim of a cereal bowl to cut out the 6-inch circles.

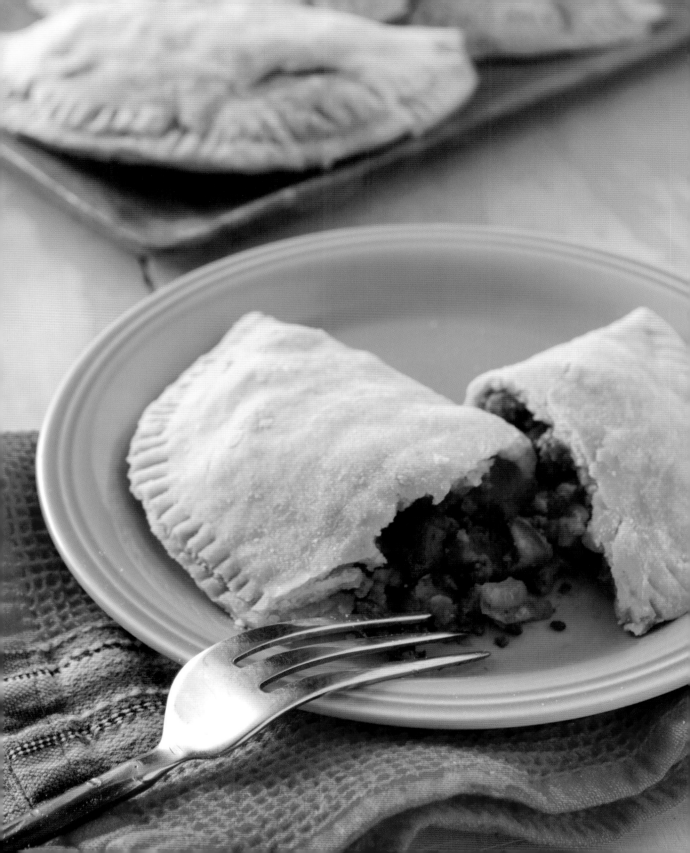

Corned Beef and Cabbage

I love corned beef, and I never get tired of having it with Irish soda bread (see page 134) on St. Patrick's Day. However, a funny thing about corned beef: My Irish friend, Paul, told me that no one he knew in Ireland ever ate corned beef on St Patrick's Day or really any other day. I guess that like the hamburgers I used to see in Paris, topped with a fried egg and dubbed "American burgers" (something I have never seen on menus here), this is an American dish that we decided to call "Irish." **SERVES 4–6**

1 3-pound corned beef brisket

2 ribs celery

2 medium carrots

1 large, yellow onion, cut in wedges

2 teaspoons salt

2 bay leaves

5 peppercorns

1 teaspoon mustard seeds

2 teaspoons whole coriander

1/4 teaspoon crushed red pepper flakes

1 1/2 pounds cabbage, shredded

1 pound potatoes, scrubbed and cubed

1. Place the corned beef brisket in a large stockpot with the celery, carrots, yellow onions, salt, bay leaves, peppercorns, mustard seeds, coriander, and crushed red pepper flakes. Cover the corned beef completely with water, plus 1 inch. Place the stockpot over medium-high heat and bring the water to a boil, reduce to a simmer, and cover. Simmer, covered, for 2 1/2 hours.

2. Using tongs, remove the vegetables from the pot and discard. Then remove the corned beef from the pot and strain the stock into another large pot in order to remove the seeds and bay leaves. Do not discard the drained stock.

3. Return the strained stock and the corned beef to the stockpot. Add the shredded cabbage and potatoes; return the stock to a boil and then reduce it to a simmer. Cover the pot and simmer for 30 minutes or until the potatoes are tender.

4. Using a slotted spoon, transfer the cabbage and potatoes from the stockpot to a large serving bowl. Remove the corned beef from the stock to a serving platter and slice it thinly, on the diagonal, against the grain of the meat.

5. Leftovers may be stored in an airtight container, refrigerated, for up to 3 days.

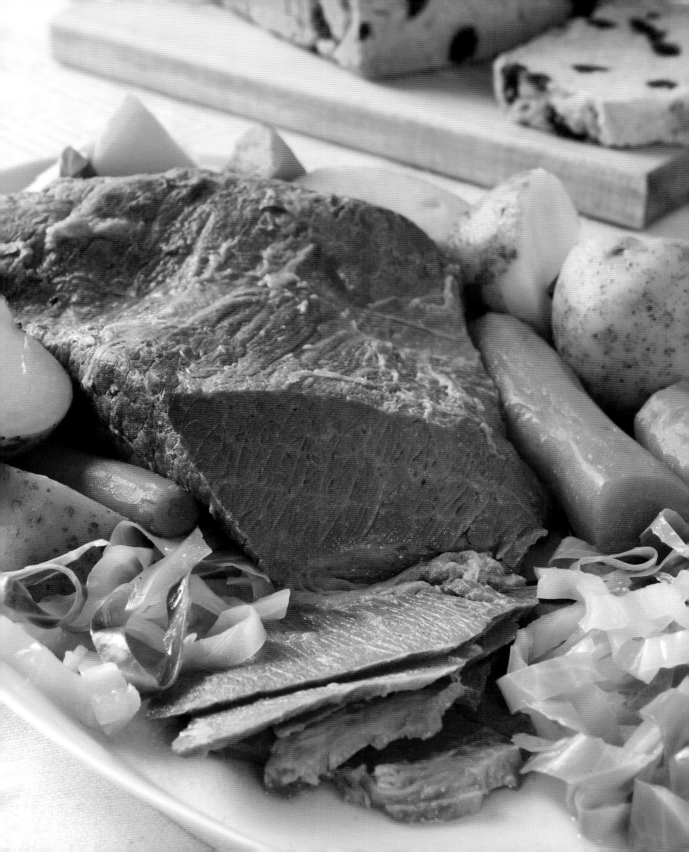

Stuffed Peppers

This is such an easy weeknight dinner, and the greatest thing about it is that you can make the peppers ahead of time and pop them in the oven when you get home from work. I love that just one pepper gives you protein, starch, and plenty of vegetables for a meal. But, the best thing about these peppers is the way my husband gobbles them up whether they are fresh from the oven or leftover from the night before. He claims to love leftovers but rarely eats them. I know I've stumbled upon a great recipe when he'll eat something the day after. SERVES 6

2 tablespoons olive oil

2 cloves garlic, minced

1 small onion, diced

1 pound ground sirloin

1½ teaspoons Italian seasoning

1 teaspoon salt

½ teaspoon black pepper

1½ cups cooked white or brown rice

1 cup canned diced tomatoes, drained

6 medium red bell peppers, tops sliced off and ribs and seeds removed

1¾ cups tomato sauce

1. Preheat the oven to 350°F.

2. In a large skillet heat the oil over medium-high heat. Add the garlic and onions and sauté until they are soft and translucent, about 3 minutes. Add the meat, breaking it up with a wooden spoon as it cooks. Continue cooking until the meat is cooked through.

3. Remove the skillet from the heat and pour off any excess fat from the pan. Stir in the Italian seasoning, salt, and pepper. Fold in the rice and the drained diced tomatoes.

4. Spoon about ¾ cup of the mixture into each of the peppers and place the peppers, upright, in a Dutch oven or a large pot fitted with a lid. Cover the peppers with the tomato sauce, cover the pot, and bake for 50 minutes or until the peppers begin to soften.

5. Leftovers may be stored in an airtight container, covered, for up to 3 days.

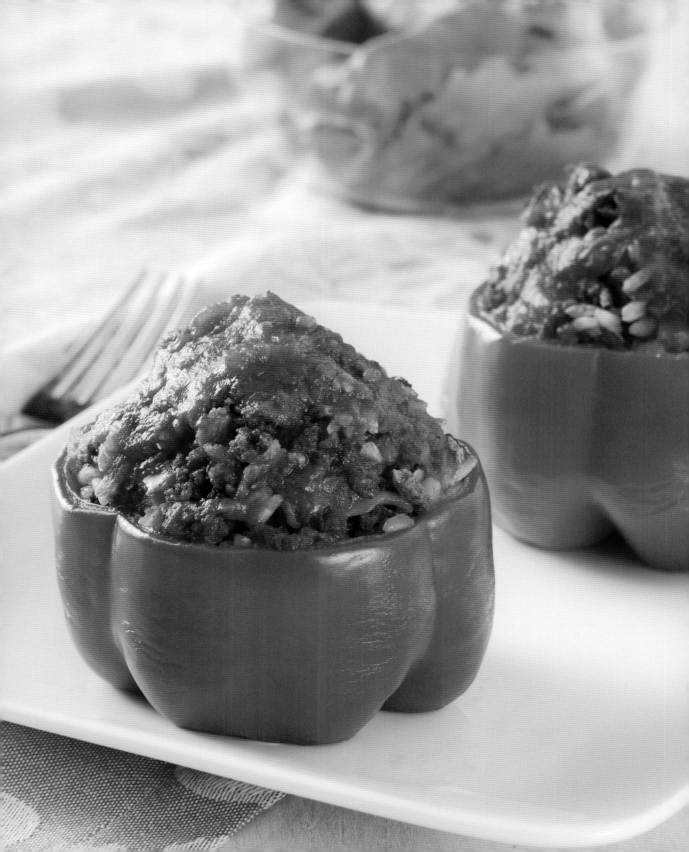

Weeknight Turkey Chili

I've said it once, and I'll say it again: I love to serve easy food during the week. Hence, I love chili. I can sneak in lots of vegetables, healthy protein, and high-fiber beans with this chili, and my family eagerly gobbles it up. The best part about this recipe is that I can make a batch and then use the leftovers to make nachos (page 38) or another dinner later in the week. Sometimes I even take the extra up to my neighbors. They love it when I bring this because they enjoy getting an entire day's worth of vegetables in one healthy bowlful. MAKES 8 1-CUP SERVINGS

1. In a large skillet brown the turkey over medium-high heat, breaking it up as you cook it. When the turkey is crumbled and cooked through, drain off the excess fat and remove it to a platter. Cover loosely with foil to keep warm; set aside.

2. Wipe out the inside of the skillet and add the olive oil. Heat the olive oil over medium-high heat. Add the onions and garlic and cook until they soften, about 2 to 3 minutes. Add the zucchini and diced peppers and sauté until they are soft, about 8 minutes. Stir in the salt, chili powder, cumin, oregano, paprika, basil, and sugar. Add the diced tomatoes and beans; bring the chili just to a simmer. Fold in the turkey and cook for another 1 to 2 minutes or until the turkey is heated through.

3. Remove the chili from the heat and serve on top of the rice. Garnish with avocado, scallions, or the toppings of your choice. Leftovers may be stored, refrigerated, in an airtight container for up to 3 days, or completely cooled chili may be frozen in airtight containers for up to 3 months.

1 pound ground turkey
1 tablespoon olive oil
1 cup diced yellow onions
    (about ¾ large)
1 clove garlic, minced
1 cup diced zucchini (about 1
    small)
1 cup diced red bell pepper
    (about 1 small), seeds and
    ribs removed
1 cup diced yellow bell pepper
    (about 1 small), seeds and
    ribs removed
2½ teaspoons salt
2 tablespoons chili powder
1 teaspoon cumin
1 teaspoon dried oregano
1 teaspoon paprika
1 teaspoon basil
1 teaspoon sugar
1 28-ounce can diced tomatoes
    in juice
1 15-ounce can kidney beans,
    rinsed and drained
1 15-ounce can black beans,
    rinsed and drained
White rice for serving
1 avocado, seeded and cubed
    (optional)
1 bunch scallions, dark
    green parts only, chopped
    (optional)

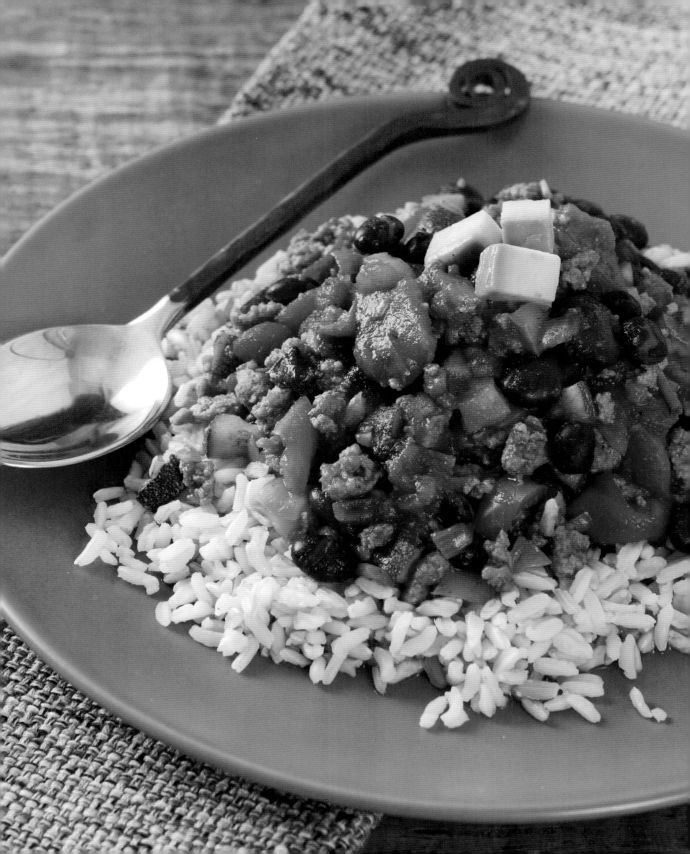

Chicken Curry

Did you know that most curry powders that you find in the supermarket do not even contain curry leaves and that most traditional Indian curries don't either? To be sure, there are some regions of India that actually include curry leaves in their stews, but for the most part, the term *curry* refers to an Indian stew made with a blend of spices that usually includes cumin, cardamom, turmeric, and sometimes cinnamon. As a cook, I'm embarrassed to admit that I not only didn't know this, but I also never took the time to flip over the bottle of curry powder to see that there was no curry leaf in it! Whether it's a blend or one spice doesn't really matter to me. I just like to eat curry, and I suppose that it is true that one learns something new every day. I especially love to make this chicken curry on a chilly night and invite a bunch of friends to dinner. SERVES 8

1¼ pounds new potatoes, scrubbed and halved

Pinch of salt

1½ teaspoons ground fennel (anise) seeds

2 teaspoons ground coriander

1 teaspoon cumin

¼ teaspoon ground cardamom

2 teaspoons turmeric

½ teaspoon ground cayenne pepper

⅛ teaspoon ground cloves

¼ teaspoon ground cinnamon

1 teaspoon salt

1 tablespoon olive oil

1 small yellow onion, cut into wedges and broken up

1 2-inch piece gingerroot, peeled and minced

1½ pounds boneless, skinless chicken breast, cubed

2½ cups canned coconut milk (lite or regular)

1 10-ounce package frozen, chopped spinach, thawed and squeezed of excess liquid

Cooked basmati rice for serving

½ cup chopped cilantro leaves

1. Place the potatoes in a large pan and cover with water, adding a generous pinch of salt. Bring the water to a boil and cook until the potatoes are tender, about 20 minutes. Drain the potatoes and set aside until you are ready to use them.

2. While the potatoes are cooking, combine the spices and salt in a small bowl. Set them aside until you are ready to use them.

3. In a large sauté pan, heat the olive oil over medium-high heat and sauté the broken-up onion wedges until they begin to soften, about 3 to 5 minutes. If the onions begin to brown, turn the heat down to medium. Add the ginger and cook another 3 to 5 minutes.

4. Pour the curry spices over the onions and ginger, stir to coat, and then add the chicken. Brown the chicken for 2 minutes; then pour in the coconut milk and stir in the spinach.

5. Bring the coconut milk just to a boil and then immediately reduce the heat to a simmer. Simmer the curry until the chicken is cooked through but tender and the sauce has started to thicken, about 12 to 15 minutes. Stir in the potatoes.

6. Serve the curry over basmati rice, sprinkled with cilantro leaves.

7. Store leftovers in an airtight container, refrigerated, for up to 3 days.

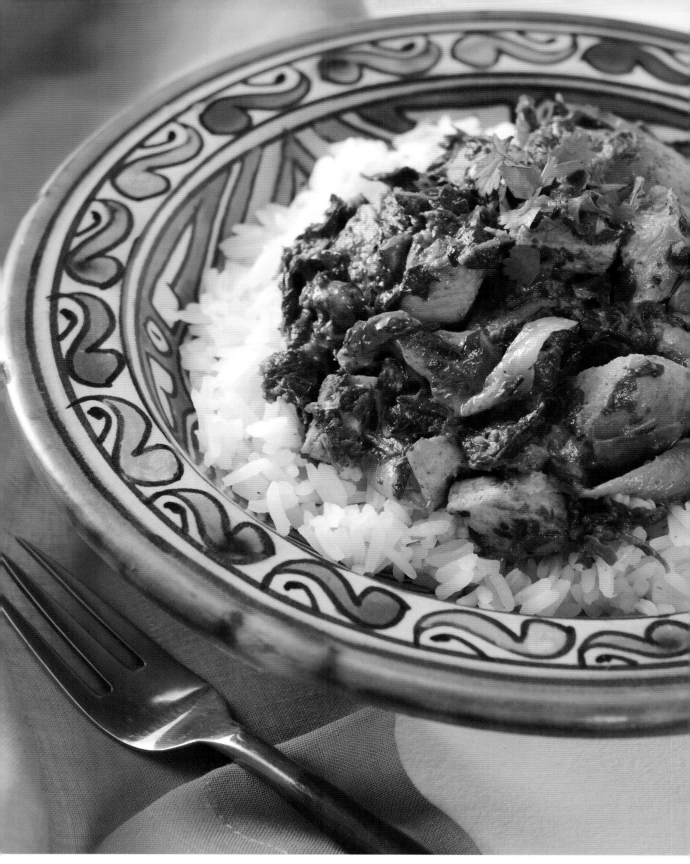

Individual Chicken Potpies

I still remember the first time I ever ate chicken potpie. Like many other first time food experiences, I was at a friend's house and didn't have a choice but to eat what her mother served me. Now, normally, at seven years old, I was ultrapicky and never would have eaten such a dish at home. However, forced into tasting this, I was surprised to find that I really loved chicken potpie. In fact I loved it so much that I used to beg my mother to let me have it on the nights that she and my father were going out. I still love it today, and this is the allergy-free version that I serve now.

SERVES 6

1 Basic Double Piecrust (see page 161)
2 tablespoons olive oil, divided
1 small yellow onion, diced
1 large clove garlic, minced
1 rib celery, diced
1 large carrot, diced
1 medium parsnip, diced
1 small zucchini, diced
1 tablespoon plus 1 teaspoon cornstarch
2 cups chicken stock (page 112), cold, divided
1/2 cup dry white wine
1/4 cup Dijon mustard
2 cups cooked chicken, diced
1/2 teaspoon salt
Dash pepper
1 teaspoon fresh thyme leaves
1 tablespoon minced Italian parsley
1 cup frozen peas, thawed
Canola oil for misting (see Where to Shop for mister recommendations)

1. Preheat the oven to 400°F.

2. Roll out the prepared dough and cut it to fit 6 4-inch mini pie plates (or roll it out and fit it into 1 9-inch pie plate). Return the prepared pie plates and the unused dough for the top layer to the refrigerator until ready to use.

3. In a large skillet heat 1 tablespoon of olive oil over medium heat and sauté the onion and garlic until they are translucent, about 5 to 7 minutes. Add the celery, carrots, parsnips, and zucchini and continue cooking until all the vegetables have softened, about another 8 minutes. Remove the vegetables to a plate.

4. In a cup whisk together the cornstarch and 1/4 cup of the cold stock; set aside.

5. In the skillet whisk together the remaining stock, wine, and remaining olive oil. Bring the mixture to a boil and slowly whisk in the cornstarch mixture. Cook for 1 minute, whisking continuously. Whisk in the Dijon mustard and simmer for another minute.

6. Remove the mixture from the heat and stir in the chicken, salt, pepper, herbs, and thawed peas.

7. Spoon the mixture into the prepared crusts. Top the potpies with the second crust, crimp the edges with a fork, and spray the tops with a little canola oil. Bake the potpies for 20 minutes or until they are golden. Store leftovers, refrigerated in an airtight container, for up to 3 days. To store unbaked pie in the freezer, allow the filling to cool completely before covering with the top crust, then wrap in plastic wrap and store in an airtight container in the freezer for up to 3 months.

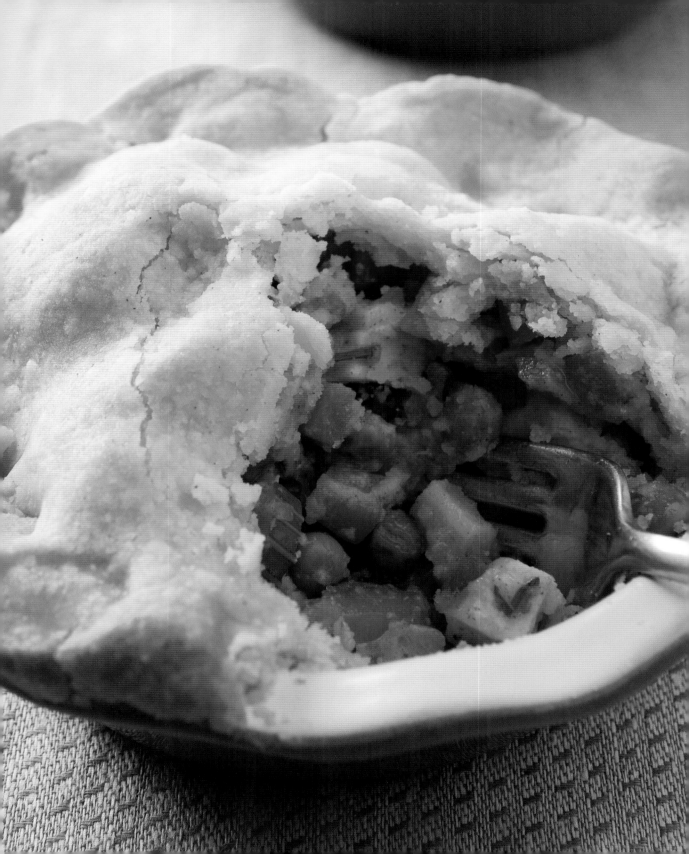

Turkey, Red Pepper, Arugula, and Hominy Soup

The name of this one says it all, for that's all that's in here. But the flavors come together to make something tasty and cozy that is perfect for curling up in front of the fire on a cold and rainy day. I love making this soup after Thanksgiving to use up all of the leftovers. This is an allergy-free twist on the classic chicken or turkey noodle soup, and with the pepper and arugula, it is packed with vitamin C to cure what ails you. SERVES 8

2 teaspoons olive oil
¼ cup chopped yellow onions
   (about ½ small onion)
1 large red bell pepper, diced
1 teaspoon salt
8 cups chicken or turkey stock
1 bunch arugula, well washed
   and leaves chopped
2 15-ounce cans hominy,
   drained
12 ounces shredded cooked
   roast turkey

1. Heat the oil in a large stockpot and cook the onions until they are translucent, about 7 minutes. Add the diced red peppers and cook until they soften, about 5 to 7 more minutes. Add the salt and stir.

2. Add the stock and bring the soup to a boil.

3. Add the chopped arugula and turn the heat down to a simmer. Simmer the soup for 5 minutes or until the arugula is completely wilted.

4. Stir in the hominy and shredded turkey. Remove the soup from the heat and serve it immediately.

5. Store leftovers in an airtight container, refrigerated, for up to 5 days. Alternately, store the completely cooled soup in airtight containers, frozen, for up to 3 months.

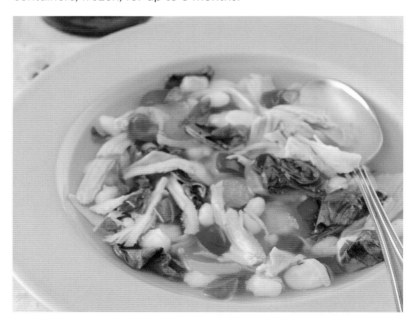

Lemon Rosemary Chicken Breasts

Sometimes you just want something quick and easy for a weeknight dinner, and this dish fits the bill. All you need are a few chicken breasts, a lemon, some rosemary, thirty minutes, and voilà, dinner is served. SERVES 4

1. Preheat the oven to 400°F and lightly grease the bottom of a 9 x 13-inch baking dish.

2. Place the chicken breasts in the greased pan and sprinkle with the chopped rosemary and salt. Place the lemon slices on top of the chicken breasts and the onion wedges around. Tightly cover the top of the baking dish with aluminum foil and bake the chicken in the preheated oven for 30 minutes.

3. When the chicken is done, remove the lemon slices and serve the chicken with the onions over the cooked rice.

4. Store leftovers in an airtight container, refrigerated, for up to 2 days.

4 boneless, skinless chicken breast halves
1/2 teaspoon chopped fresh rosemary
1/2 teaspoon salt
1 small lemon, thinly sliced
1 large yellow onion, cut in wedges
Cooked brown rice for serving

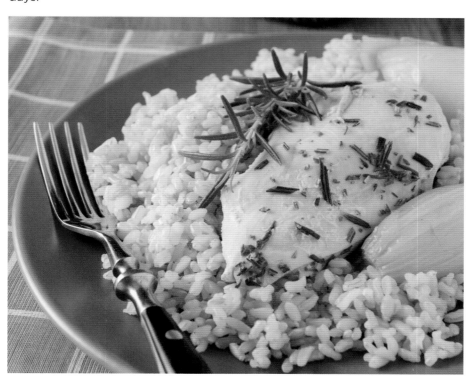

Chicken Soft Tacos

Every Sunday night on our way back into the city, we inevitably stop at a little place in Southold, New York, called the Rotisserie. Honestly, they make the best duck legs and chicken soft tacos I have ever tasted, and their spicy sauce inspired my Spicy Tomatillo Sauce (page 65). Whenever we go, I get the chicken soft tacos, and it was from this restaurant's style of serving tacos that I learned you don't need a crunchy shell, cheese, and sour cream, just really fresh ingredients, to make a taco taste good. This is my version of the Rotisserie's chicken soft taco. Serve it with my Spicy Tomatillo Sauce to get the full effect. SERVES 4

2 teaspoons olive oil
1 pound ground chicken
1/2 teaspoon salt
1 teaspoon cumin
Generous pinch cayenne
  pepper
1/4 cup chopped cilantro, plus
  additional for garnish
2 teaspoons lime zest
Dash black pepper
8 6-inch corn tortillas
1/2 pint cherry tomatoes, cut
  into thirds
1/4 large red onion, diced
Spicy Tomatillo Sauce (see
  page 65) (optional)

1. Heat the oil in a large skillet over medium-high heat.

2. In a large bowl mix together the ground chicken, salt, cumin, cayenne pepper, cilantro, and lime zest.

3. Cook the chicken mixture in the hot oil, breaking it up with a wooden spoon as it cooks, for about 10 minutes or until the chicken is cooked through. Stir in the pepper.

4. Just before the chicken is done cooking, heat the corn tortillas over the open flame of a gas burner, if possible. Place one tortilla over a low flame, turning it with tongs until it appears to "wilt," after about 30 seconds. Or, you may also wrap the tortillas in a damp paper towel and microwave for 45 seconds or until they are warm and pliable.

5. Distribute the cooked chicken mixture among the warmed tortillas and spoon on some tomatoes and red onion. Serve with Spicy Tomatillo Sauce if desired. Serve immediately.

6. The leftover meat filling may be stored in an airtight container, refrigerated, for up to 3 days.

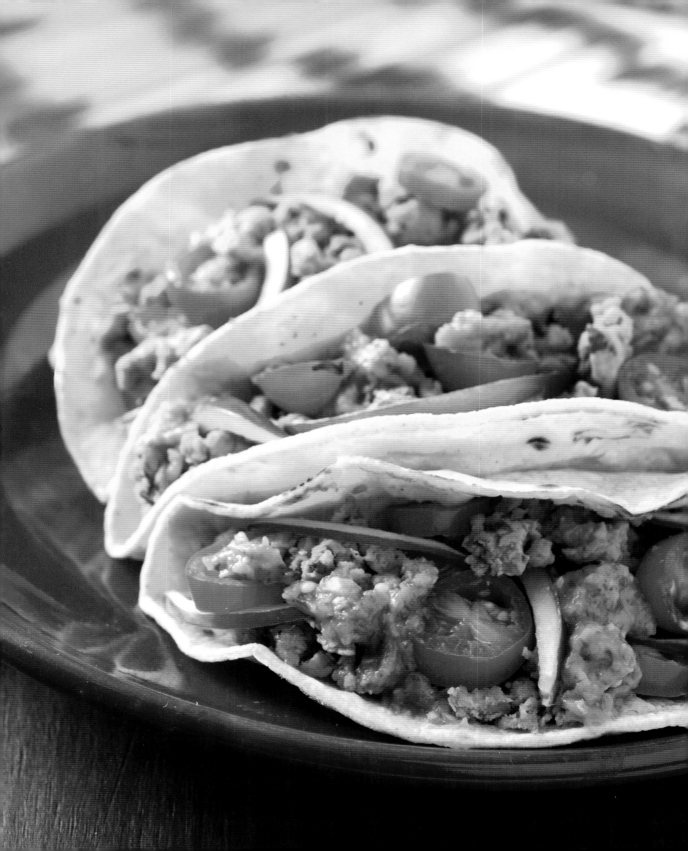

Fried Chicken

To me, fried chicken is the taste of summer. Before I was diagnosed with food allergies, we used to pick up big boxes of fried chicken and donuts and have wonderful lunchtime beach picnics. All of that ended when I learned that wheat and eggs were out. So when I started playing around with gluten-, dairy-, soy-, nut-, and egg-free savory dishes, this was one of the first things I made. While deep-frying chicken isn't the healthiest way to cook it, I consider this a treat and eat it in moderation. The crispy coating is so flavorful and crunchy, and the chicken inside so moist and delicious. The key to this delicious chicken is the double coating of breading, never skimp on that step. I think it just might have been worth the six-year wait. SERVES 6

2 cups rice milk
2 tablespoons cider vinegar
3 pounds bone-in, quartered
   chicken pieces
1 recipe All-Purpose Breading
   (see page 66)
Canola oil for frying

1. In a large shallow bowl, whisk together the rice milk and vinegar. Place the chicken pieces in the bowl so that they are covered, cover the bowl, and put it in the refrigerator. Let the chicken soak for 3 hours.

2. While the chicken is soaking, prepare the All-Purpose Breading according to the recipe directions and pour it into a large shallow bowl.

3. Fill a fryer with canola oil according to the fryer instructions. If you are using a skillet, fill it with 3 to 4 inches of canola oil. Preheat the fryer or oil in the skillet to 350°F.

4. When the chicken is finished soaking, remove it from the refrigerator and, working one piece at a time, dip it in the All-Purpose Breading until it is completely but lightly coated, return it to the rice milk mixture, and then coat it one more time in the All-Purpose Breading mix.

5. Fry the coated chicken in the preheated oil for 7 minutes per piece, carefully turning occasionally with tongs, careful not to overcrowd the fryer. Remove the finished chicken to paper towel–lined plates to drain.

6. If you prefer to bake the chicken instead of frying it, preheat the oven to 400°F and place the coated chicken on a lightly oiled, rimmed baking sheet. Bake the chicken for 45 minutes, flipping the pieces after 25 minutes. Serve immediately.

7. Although the chicken is best enjoyed at once, uneaten pieces may be stored in airtight containers, refrigerated, for up to 3 days.

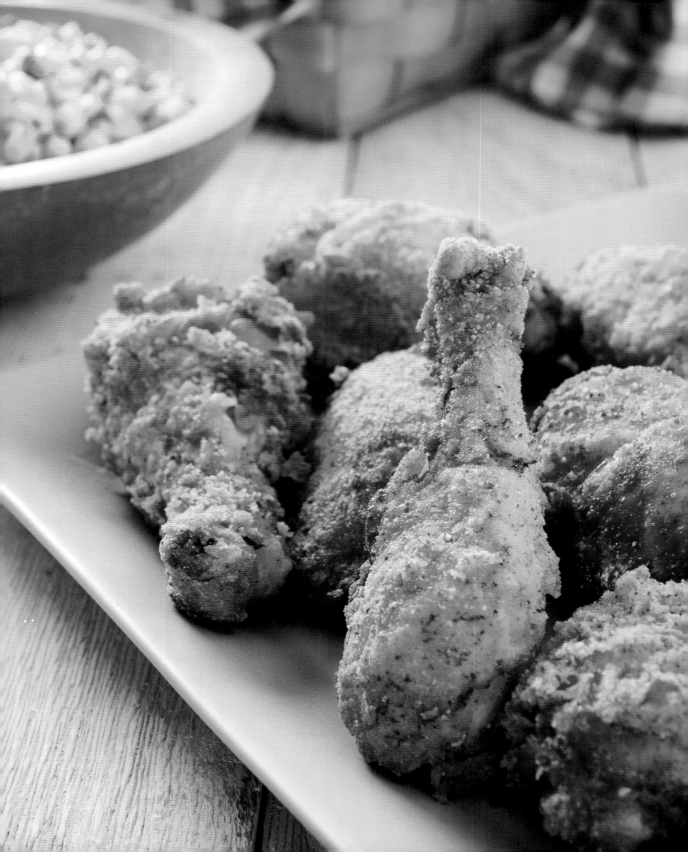

Perfect Roast Chicken

Roast chicken is supposed to be one of the easiest dinners to make, and yet I find it difficult. When the chicken is whole and stuffed, it is very hard to get the cooking time just right so that the chicken is completely cooked but the breast isn't dry. I found a few years ago that the easiest, fastest, and most sure-fire way to a perfect whole chicken is to butterfly it. The chicken cooks faster but evenly and is never dry. I like this method so much that I even cook my Thanksgiving turkey this way! SERVES 4–6

1 3-pound whole chicken, washed and patted dry
2 tablespoons olive oil, divided
1/2 teaspoon salt, divided
2 large parsnips, peeled and sliced 1/4 inch thick
3 large carrots, peeled and sliced 1/4 inch thick
1 pound new potatoes, scrubbed and quartered
Dash pepper

1. Preheat the oven to 425°F.

2. Using poultry shears, cut up one side of the chicken's spine and down the other. Discard the spine. Flip the chicken over so that the breast side is up and press down firmly on the breast bone to break it, flattening the chicken. Place the chicken in a roasting pan (I like to use a large paella pan); rub it with 2 teaspoons olive oil and 1/4 teaspoon salt.

3. Mix together the remaining olive oil, parsnips, carrots, potatoes, remaining 1/4 teaspoon salt, and pepper until the vegetables are well coated. Dump the vegetables out into the roasting pan and arrange them around the chicken. Place the roasting pan in the preheated oven and roast for 1 hour.

4. Remove the chicken from the oven and pierce the thickest part of the thigh with a knife, checking to be sure that the juices run clear, or use an instant-read thermometer to be sure that the internal temperature is 165°F in the breast.

5. Let the chicken rest for 10 minutes before slicing. Toss the roasted vegetables with the pan juices before serving.

6. Leftovers may be stored in an airtight container, refrigerated, for up to 3 days.

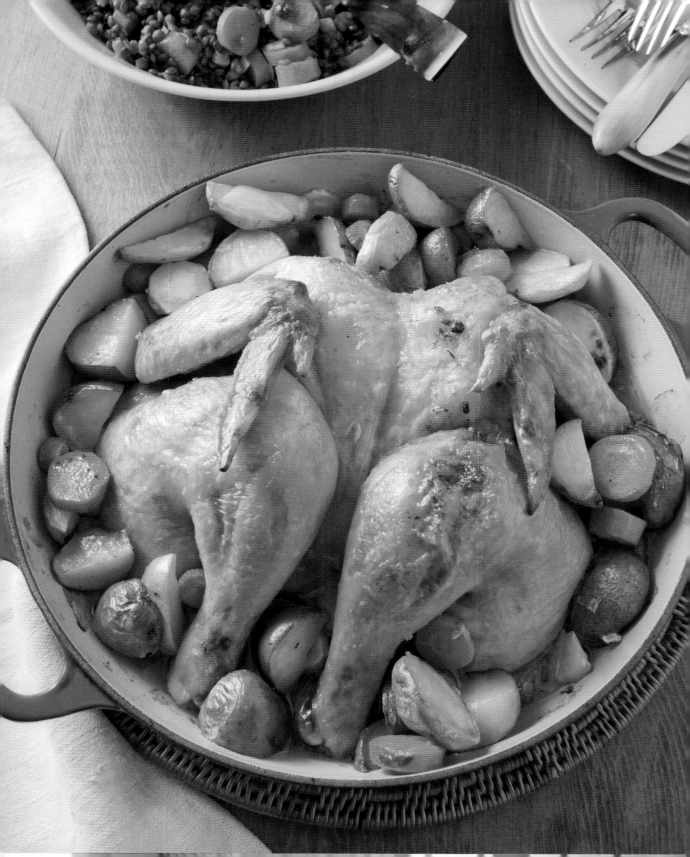

Pizza

A few years ago, I met with a nutritionist to go over my diet and to find ways to improve it. She told me that she actually loves pizza because it is a complete meal. I always thought of pizza as junk food, but then I realized that she was right—especially when you make it yourself and it's less greasy. The crust is a healthy carbohydrate, and when I make pizza, it is loaded with vegetables. The possibilities are endless, and this, in my opinion, is the best thing about pizza. Go crazy with the vegetables on top. Add olives or herbs. Any way you slice it, it's a great dinner that your entire family will love. SERVES 4-6

Crust
1 recipe All-Purpose Savory Pastry (see page 67)
Cornmeal for dusting the pizza pan

Suggested Toppings
Tomato sauce (I like Muir Glen Pizza Sauce) or roasted cherry tomatoes, artichokes, sliced black olives, cooked broccoli, sliced and cooked zucchini, soy-free ham or cooked bacon if you are not interested in making it a vegetarian meal, roasted garlic, dairy- and soy-free Daiya cheese or the allergy-friendly cheese of your choice, freshly torn basil leaves, red pepper flakes, oregano

1. Preheat the oven to 425°F and lightly sprinkle a 16-inch pizza pan with the cornmeal. Prepare the pastry dough according to the recipe directions. Press the dough out so that it is thin in the center but you can turn over the edges to create a traditional pizza crust.

2. When the dough is formed into the shape of a pizza, place it in the preheated oven and bake for 12 minutes. Remove the crust from the oven; top it with ½ cup of sauce and whatever other toppings you like. Return the pizza to the oven and bake for an additional 12 minutes.

3. Remove the pizza from the oven and let it cool 5 minutes before cutting it. Serve immediately.

4. Store leftovers in an airtight container, refrigerated, for up to 3 days.

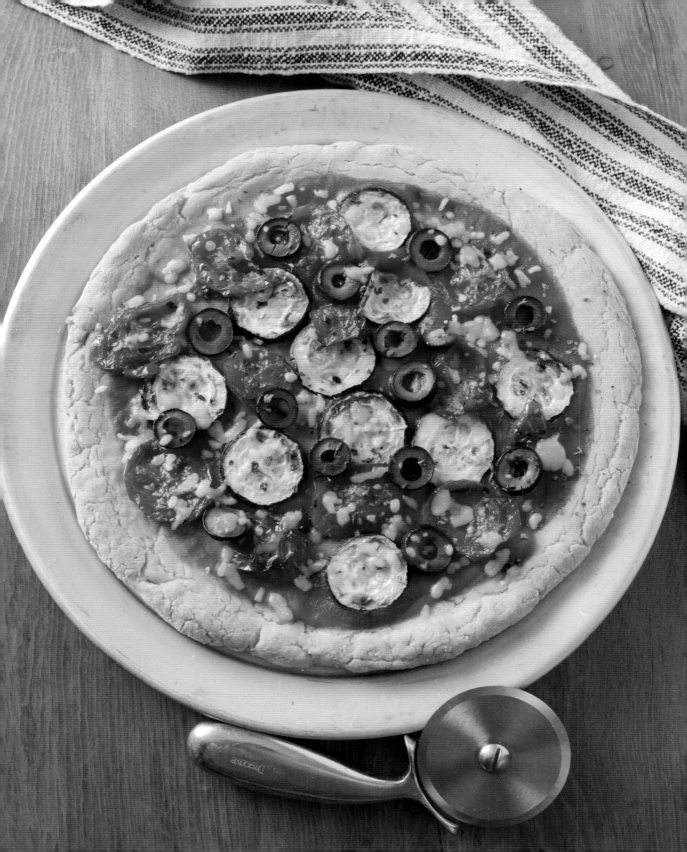

Pupusas

When I tell my children that I'm making pupusas, they actually cheer. Pupusas are quick to make and take the place of grilled cheese or panini in our household; I generally have the ingredients around, and my kids always say yes to helping with the preparations. I make up batches of bean pupusas and keep them in the freezer for a quick lunch. Pupusas are an El Salvadoran street food, and we started eating them a few years ago when a friend of El Salvadoran descent introduced us to them. They were an instant Gordon family classic. If you aren't vegetarian, stuff the pupusas with leftover barbecue pork from my Shredded Pork Sandwiches (see page 88) instead. MAKES 16 PUPUSAS

2 cups masa harina corn flour, not cornmeal (see Where to Shop)

2 cups plus 2 tablespoons water

Canola oil, as needed

1 cup vegetarian soy-free refried beans or Daiya cheese

Cubed avocado, salsa, or shredded cabbage for serving, optional

1. In a large mixing bowl, combine the masa harina and water with your fingers. It should form a dough that is not thin and watery, but thick and moist. Press plastic wrap directly on top of the dough and let it sit for 5 minutes.

2. Very lightly oil a griddle with canola oil and then preheat the griddle over medium-high heat.

3. While the griddle is heating, form the pupusas. With wet hands, roll 2 tablespoons of the dough between your hands to form a ball. Poke a hole about a quarter of the way through the ball with your thumb. Press 1 to 2 teaspoons of the cheese or beans (or both) into the hole, and form the dough around the filling until it is a ball again. Then, pat the pupusa between your palms until it is flat like a pancake. The edges of the pupusas should be smooth. If the edges crack or look dry, add 1 to 2 tablespoons water to the dough.

4. Place the pupusas on the heated griddle and cook over medium-high heat for 7 to 8 minutes per side. Continue rolling and stuffing the pupusas until all the dough is used.

5. Serve immediately with avocado, salsa, or, more traditionally, shredded cabbage.

6. Leftovers can be stored in an airtight container for up to 3 days. Or you can place completely cooled pupusas in an airtight container with squares of waxed paper between each one and freeze for up to 3 months. To reheat frozen puposas, preheat the oven to 400°F. Place puposas on a rimmed baking sheet and bake for 10 to 15 minutes or until warmed through. Serve immediately.

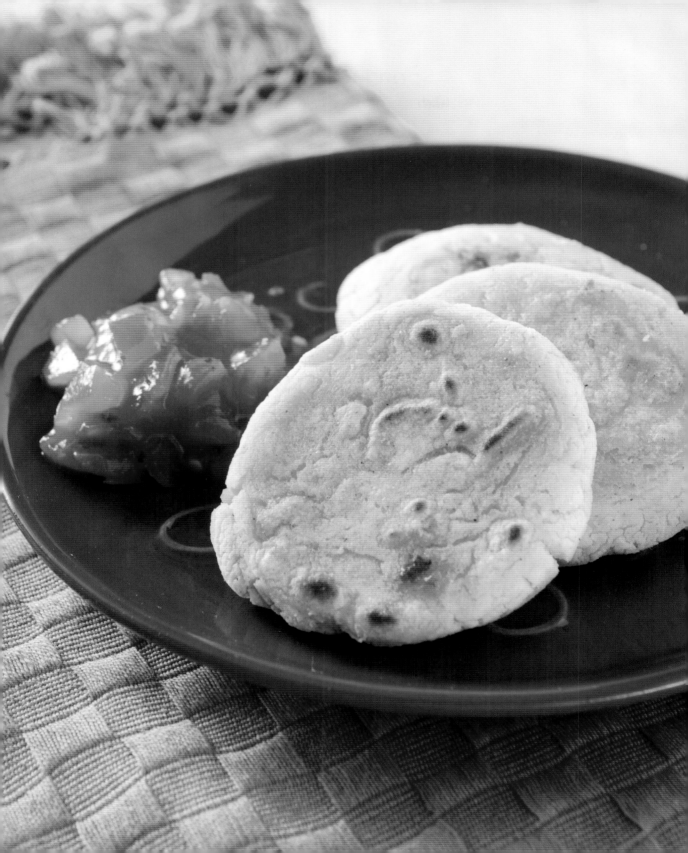

Spring Risotto

We are huge fans of risotto. Though this version is loaded with green spring vegetables, there is no reason your risotto can't contain any number of other ingredients. Use this recipe as a basic starting point and then add whatever vegetables you have in your refrigerator, sautéed. Or, omit all the vegetables and just add a handful of herbs and a little lemon zest. If you are not vegetarian, you could also make this recipe with some leeks and a handful of crisp bacon sprinkled on top. With one recipe and a little imagination, you can easily make a month's worth of simple dinners.

SERVES 4

3 cups vegetable stock
2 tablespoons olive oil
1 clove garlic, minced
1 very small yellow onion, diced
1 cup Arborio rice
½ cup white cooking wine
¾ teaspoon marjoram
½ teaspoon salt
1 10-ounce package frozen spinach, thawed and squeezed of excess moisture
1 cup frozen peas, thawed
1 tablespoon soy- and dairy-free margarine

1. Pour the stock into a medium saucepan and heat over medium heat until it just simmers. Turn the heat down to low.

2. Meanwhile, in a large sauté pan, heat the oil over medium-high heat. When the oil is hot, add in the garlic and onions and cook until they are soft and translucent, about 5 to 7 minutes.

3. Add the Arborio rice and stir to coat it with the olive oil. Let the rice cook in the hot oil for about 30 seconds to open the grains. Pour in the wine, stir the rice, and let it cook for another 30 seconds to cook off the alcohol. Turn the heat down to medium.

4. Add 2 cups of the warmed stock and stir the rice until the stock is completely absorbed. Add the remaining stock a half cup at a time, stirring after each addition until all of the stock is absorbed and the rice is soft, about 20 minutes. Stir in the marjoram, salt, vegetables, and margarine and serve.

5. Leftovers can be stored in an airtight container, refrigerated, for up to 3 days.

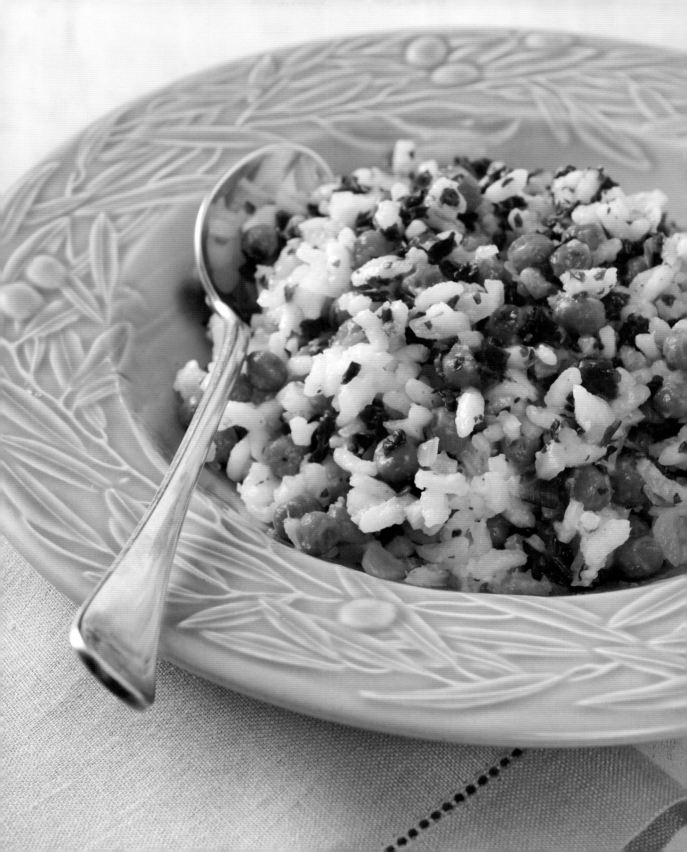

Marinara Sauce

My youngest daughter is very finicky, so it was a red-letter day when she not only agreed to try sauce on her pasta but also admitted that she liked it. In fact it felt nothing short of miraculous. Although I prefer to serve my children vegetables that are raw or just barely steamed, this sauce stands in when everyone is feeling especially persnickety. MAKES 1 QUART

2 tablespoons olive oil
1 clove garlic, minced
1 cup diced onions (about ½ large onion)
1 tablespoon red wine
1½ teaspoons salt
¼ teaspoon black pepper
1½ teaspoons Italian seasoning
1 28-ounce can whole peeled tomatoes in thick puree
⅔ cup water
1 teaspoon sugar

1. Heat the olive oil in a large saucepan over medium-high heat. Add the garlic and onions and sauté for about 8 minutes or until the onions are very soft.

2. Add the wine and let it cook off for about 30 seconds. Add the salt, pepper, and Italian seasoning and stir well.

3. Add the tomatoes, breaking them up very well with a wooden spoon.

4. Add the water and sugar and stir the sauce well. Bring the sauce to a boil, reduce the heat to a simmer, and simmer for 20 minutes.

5. Serve the sauce immediately over spaghetti squash or gluten-free pasta.

6. The leftover sauce may be stored in an airtight container, refrigerated, for up to 3 days. You can also freeze the completely cooled sauce in an airtight container for up to 3 months.

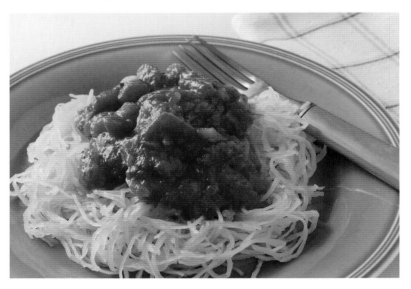

Black Beans and Yellow Rice

This is the best thing in the world to eat for lunch on a chilly afternoon. Cozy, delicious, and definitely vegetarian, the rice and beans combine to form a complete protein. Just serve it with a salad for a well-rounded meal. If you are not vegetarian, this pairs particularly well as a side dish to my Perfect Roast Chicken (see page 110). SERVES 4

1. In a medium saucepan fitted with a lid, heat the oil over medium-high heat. Add the onions and garlic and sauté until they have softened, about 3 minutes.

2. Add the rice, vegetable stock, salt, and turmeric and bring to a boil. When it begins to boil, reduce the rice to a simmer and cover the saucepan. Reduce the heat to low and simmer the rice, covered, for 20 minutes. Remove the rice from the heat and fluff it with a fork.

3. While the rice is cooking, combine the beans, cumin, and cayenne pepper in another small saucepan and heat over low heat until just heated through. Stir in the lime juice.

4. Serve the beans over the rice, sprinkled with a few cilantro leaves for garnish.

5. Leftovers may be stored in an airtight container, refrigerated, for up to 3 days.

1 tablespoon canola oil
1/4 cup diced yellow onions
1 clove garlic, minced
1 cup white rice
2 cups vegetable stock
1/2 teaspoon salt
1/2 teaspoon turmeric
1 15-ounce can black beans, rinsed and drained
3/4 teaspoon cumin
1/4 teaspoon cayenne pepper
1 teaspoon fresh lime juice
Cilantro leaves for serving

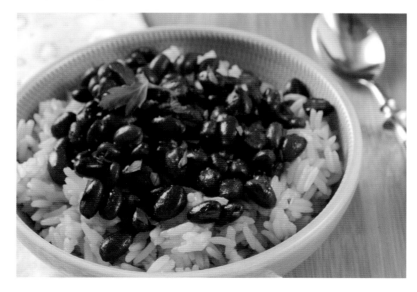

Black Bean Burgers

A few years ago my friend decided to go vegan. She came to visit us for a weekend, and I wanted to make something that all of us liked to eat. Since I had planned on making burgers for the carnivores, I didn't want her to feel left out of the fun. At the end of all the cooking, I actually opted for my black bean burgers over the regular burgers. Spicy and with just the right texture, they are delicious with or without a gluten-free bun. The best part is that they are not bound with egg like so many veggie burgers sold in the freezer section. SERVES 6

1 16-ounce can black beans, drained and rinsed

3 cloves garlic, minced

$\frac{1}{2}$ medium onion, diced

2 ribs celery, diced

1 teaspoon dry mustard

$\frac{1}{2}$ teaspoon salt

3 tablespoons tomato paste

1 teaspoon cornstarch

1$\frac{1}{4}$ teaspoon chili powder

1 teaspoon cumin

Dash Tabasco (optional)

1 cup cooked brown or white rice

$\frac{1}{2}$ cup ground flaxseed meal

2 tablespoons olive oil

Avocado slices and diced fresh tomatoes for serving

1. Preheat the oven to 350°F and very lightly grease a rimmed baking sheet.

2. In a large bowl mash $\frac{3}{4}$ cup of the black beans with a fork. Leave the remaining beans whole.

3. Add the garlic, onions, celery, dry mustard, salt, tomato paste, cornstarch, chili powder, cumin, and Tabasco if using to the bowl of a food processor. Process until the mixture is a smooth paste.

4. Fold the paste into the cooked rice and then fold in the mashed and whole beans. Scoop the mixture with a $\frac{1}{3}$ cup measuring cup, and form it into 6 patties. Place the ground flaxseed meal in a large shallow bowl and carefully coat each patty in the flaxseed meal.

5. Heat the oil over medium-high heat in a large skillet. Place the coated patties in the heated oil and fry for 3 minutes per side.

6. After frying both sides, place the patties on the prepared baking sheet and bake them for 20 minutes. Serve topped with tomato slices and the diced avocado.

7. Although these burgers are best served immediately, they may be completely cooled and stored in an airtight container, with a square of wax paper between them if you stack them, refrigerated, for up to 3 days. Or, you may freeze them in the same fashion for up to 3 months. To reheat frozen burgers, preheat the oven to 400°F. Place burgers on a rimmed baking sheet and bake for 10 to 15 minutes or until warmed through. Serve immediately.

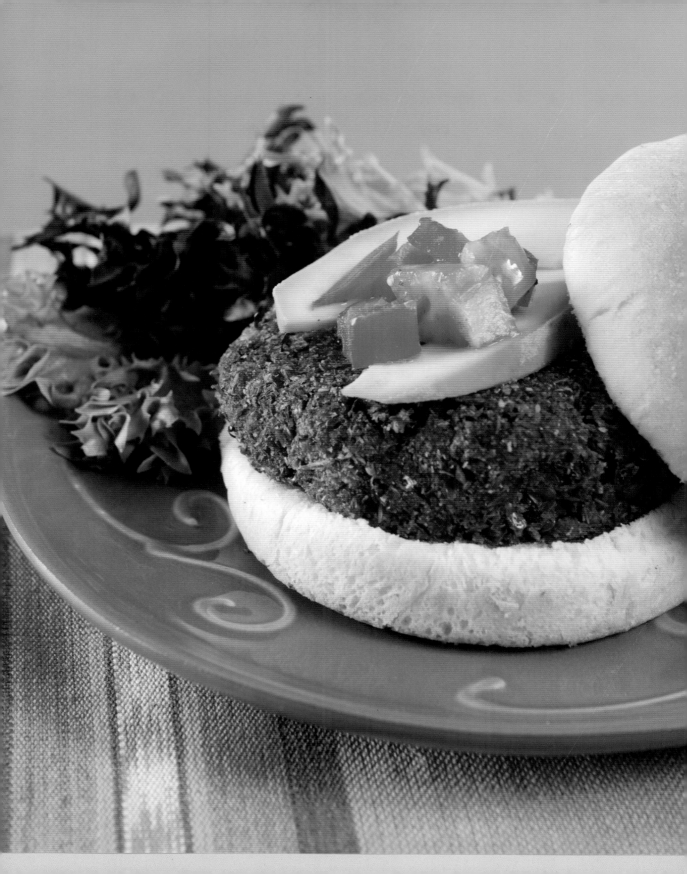

Hush Puppies

In Ohio, hush puppies were something that one only got at Long John Silver's, and as my parents never took us there to eat, I didn't eat too many hush puppies as a child. But then I went to Tennessee for high school and ate them every time we had catfish, which was often. When my good friend invited me down to North Carolina after we had graduated from college, I jumped at the chance to see her and to eat some of my Southern favorites. I have a very vivid memory of going to a peel-and-eat shrimp joint on the water one night during the visit and being thrilled when the basket of hush puppies appeared. The little balls of fried cornbread laced with tiny pieces of onion were something I had missed so much since I had gone back up north for college. The draw of the restaurant was the shrimp, but I was far more interested in the wax paper–lined baskets overflowing with hush puppies. In fact I think I skipped dinner and just had the puppies.

MAKES 22 HUSH PUPPIES

Canola oil for frying

2 cups cornmeal

3/4 cup Chinese or superfine rice flour

3 tablespoons potato starch

1 tablespoon sorghum flour

1/2 teaspoon baking soda

1 teaspoon baking powder

3/4 teaspoon salt

1/4 teaspoon paprika

1/4 teaspoon black pepper

7/8 teaspoon xanthan gum

1 cup coconut milk kefir

1 tablespoon cider vinegar

1/4 cup diced onions (about 1/2 small onion)

1. Fill a fryer with canola oil according to the fryer instructions or fill a large skillet with about 3 to 4 inches of canola oil. Preheat the fryer or skillet to 350°F.

2. In a large bowl whisk together the cornmeal, rice flour, potato starch, sorghum flour, baking soda, baking powder, salt, paprika, black pepper, and xanthan gum.

3. In a small, separate bowl, stir together the kefir and cider vinegar, then stir into the dry ingredients. Fold in the diced onions.

4. Scoop the batter with a 1 1/2-inch ice cream scoop and release the scoop into the preheated oil. Fry the hush puppies, a few at a time so as not to overcrowd the fryer, for 4 minutes, or until they are golden brown on all sides. If they stick to the bottom of the fryer basket, gently loosen them with tongs, making sure they remain intact.

5. Remove the fried hush puppies to a paper towel–lined plate to drain. Serve immediately.

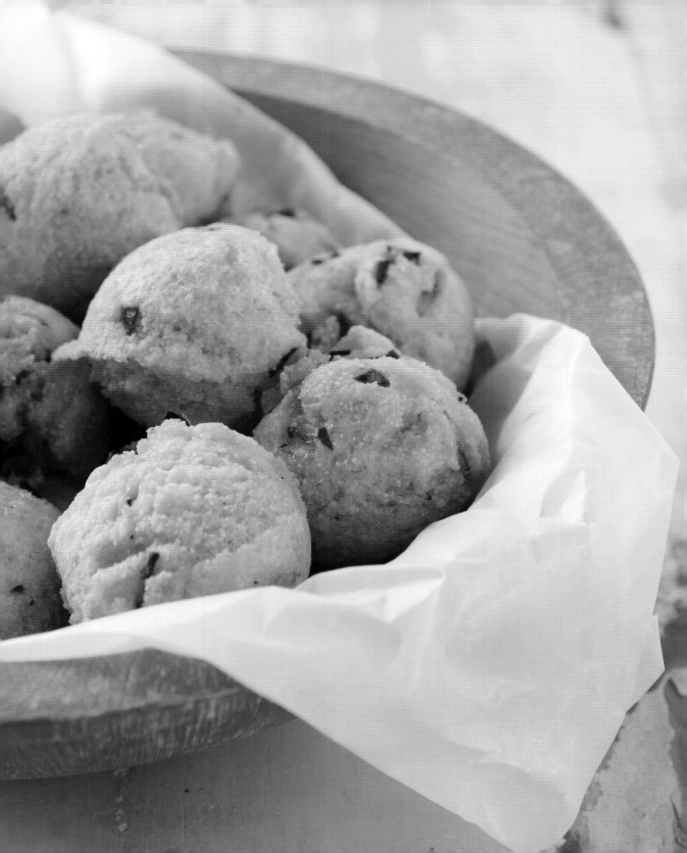

Rosemary Smashed Potatoes

Mashed potatoes were one of my favorite dishes as a child. I remember the excitement that welled up in my stomach when my mother took out the potato masher and the pink pitcher that she used exclusively for melting the milk and butter for her recipe. Luckily, even without milk and butter, mashed potatoes can still taste great. My recipe uses flavorful olive oil and aromatic rosemary to perk up this perfect mash. SERVES 5

1½ pounds red potatoes, quartered

Generous pinch of salt

¼ cup olive oil

1 clove garlic, pressed

2 teaspoons minced fresh rosemary leaves

¾ teaspoon salt

Dash pepper

1. Place the potatoes in a large pot and cover with water. Add salt to the water and bring to a boil. Boil for 15 minutes or until the potatoes are soft.

2. Drain the potatoes, return them to the pan, add the olive oil, and mash with a hand masher. Fold in the pressed garlic, rosemary, salt, and pepper. The potatoes should be lumpy, not smooth. Serve immediately.

3. Leftovers may be stored, refrigerated, in an airtight container for 3 to 5 days.

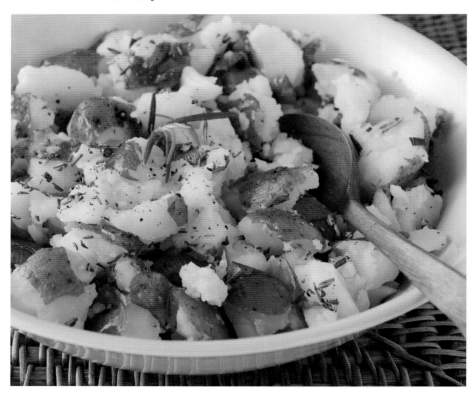

Easy Roasted Potatoes

I make roasted potatoes for our family at least once a week. They are a healthier and slightly more sophisticated alternative to french fries, and almost all of us love them. Experiment with the herbs: Try rosemary or oregano or thyme, maybe even a squeeze of lemon juice. Only your imagination can limit you. I make this recipe for large gatherings and simply halve it for weeknight dinners. **SERVES 10**

1. Preheat the oven to 400°F and prepare two or three baking sheets by lining them with parchment paper.

2. Combine the potatoes, oil, salt, pepper, garlic cloves, and rosemary in a mixing bowl until the potatoes are well coated with the oil and salt. Pour them onto the prepared baking sheets.

3. Roast the potatoes for 60 minutes or until they are golden brown all over, making sure to turn the potatoes twice while they are baking.

4. Serve immediately. Store leftovers, refrigerated, for 3 to 5 days.

Note: For easier cleanup, these potatoes are terrific made on the grill. Dump the potatoes, oil, salt, pepper, garlic, and rosemary onto sheets of aluminum foil and then fold over the edges to make tightly sealed pouches. Place the pouches on a preheated grill (400°F), cover, and cook for 40 minutes.

4 pounds new, red, or fingerling potatoes, halved
6 tablespoons olive oil
2 teaspoons coarse sea salt
1/2 teaspoon black pepper
2 garlic cloves, sliced thin
3 tablespoons finely chopped fresh rosemary

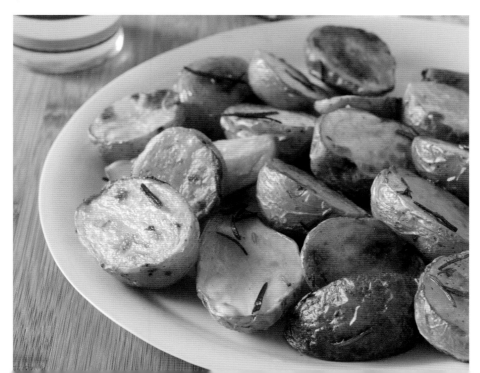

Brown Bread

This simple, yeast-free bread makes an excellent sandwich bread but also stands alone as a terrific toast. I find this recipe interesting because while the gluten-free beer does add a deep flavor to the bread, it is actually there to make the bread rise in the absence of yeast. The best part about this bread is that it is so quick and easy, and it pairs well with most anything. My favorite way to eat it is spread with a butter substitute, a sprinkle of coarse sea salt, and a slice of cucumber on top. SERVES 12

1 cup Chinese rice flour
1 cup millet flour
²/₃ cup potato starch
¹/₃ cup sorghum flour
1 tablespoon plus 1 ¹/₂ teaspoons baking powder
1 ³/₄ teaspoons salt
¹/₄ cup granulated sugar
2 ¹/₂ teaspoons xanthan gum
12 ounces sorghum (gluten-free) beer (see Where to Shop)
Ice for a water bath in the oven
3 tablespoons olive oil

1. Preheat the oven to 350°F. Lightly grease a 9 x 5-inch loaf pan with canola oil and set it aside.

2. In a large mixing bowl, whisk together the rice flour, millet flour, potato starch, sorghum flour, baking powder, salt, sugar, and xanthan gum. Pour in the sorghum beer and mix the batter with a spatula until it is thoroughly combined; the batter will look more like cake batter than bread dough. Pour the batter into the prepared pan and smooth the top with a knife.

3. Meanwhile, gather 2 cups of ice and enough cold water to fill a 9 x 13-inch metal baking pan halfway. Place the baking pan on the bottom of the oven and place the bread pan on the middle rack of the oven.

4. Bake the bread for 10 minutes. Remove the bread from the oven and, using a pastry brush, brush the top with the olive oil. Return the bread to the oven and bake for another 35 minutes or until the top is golden and a toothpick inserted in the center comes out clean.

5. Let the bread cool in the pan for 15 minutes and then turn it out onto a cooling rack to cool completely before slicing.

6. Store any leftover bread, tightly wrapped in plastic wrap, refrigerated, for up to 5 days or freeze it for up to 3 months.

Note: The water bath in the bottom of the oven is an old baking trick that keeps the bread moist while simultaneously providing even baking and browning.

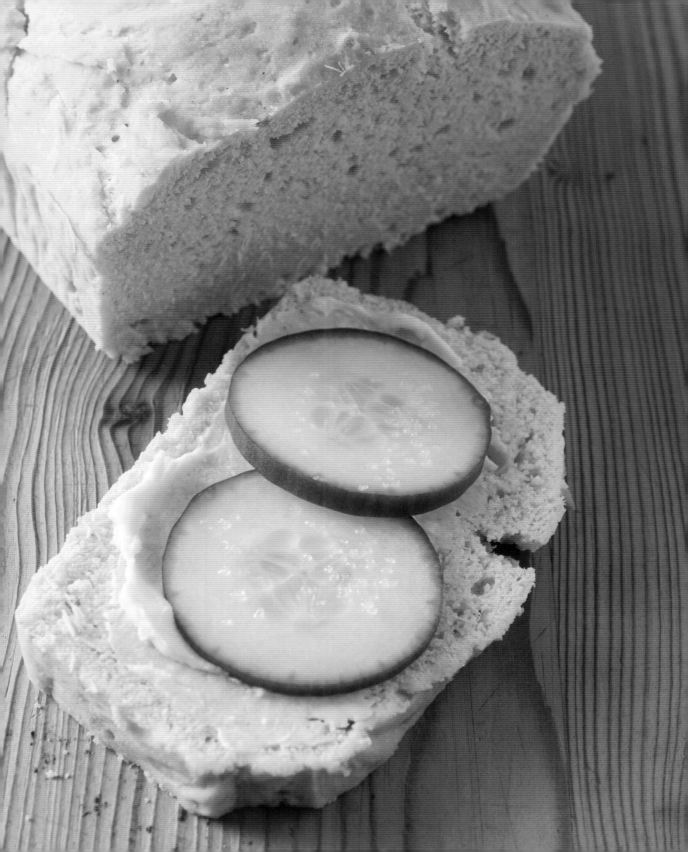

Oven-Baked Fries

Everyone I know loves a side of fries, but with my wheat allergy, I can no longer eat them at restaurants. Too many other breaded things go into the fryer with or before the french fries. Luckily, fries are easy to make at home. Occasionally I make them in the fryer, but because my girls like to eat fries often, I like to know that they are relatively low in fat and few in ingredients. This baked version crisps up nicely if baked on an unlined metal baking sheet. SERVES 4

2 pounds Russet potatoes
2 tablespoons olive oil
1 teaspoon coarse sea salt, like
   Maldon

1. Preheat the oven to 400°F.

2. Peel the potatoes and slice them, lengthwise, into fifths. Turn the potatoes on their sides and vertically slice in fifths again. This should yield the traditional french fry shape. If some of the fifths are still too wide, cut those in half.

3. Place the cut potatoes in a large ziplock bag, pour in the olive oil, seal, and shake the bag to evenly coat the fries.

4. Dump the fries onto an unlined, ungreased rimmed baking sheet, sprinkle with the salt, and bake for 40 minutes, turning after 20 minutes.

5. Serve the fries immediately.

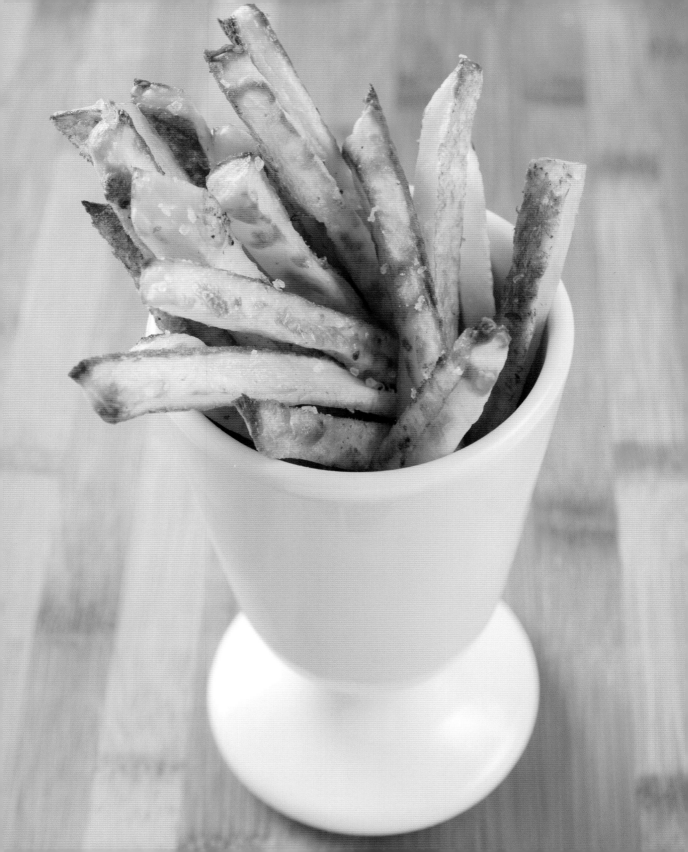

Irish Soda Bread

This is the perfect accompaniment to my corned beef and cabbage (see page 92). I love to make this both on St. Patrick's Day and for regular weekdays. It is great for breakfast with apple butter or spread with dairy- and soy-free margarine. It toasts well, so it is also delicious in my cinnamon toast (see page 21). SERVES 12

2 cups Chinese or superfine rice flour

²/₃ cup potato starch

¹/₃ cup sorghum flour

2 ¹/₂ teaspoons xanthan gum

1 teaspoon salt

1 tablespoon baking powder

1 teaspoon baking soda

¹/₃ cup granulated sugar

¹/₄ cup unsweetened applesauce

2 cups So Delicious coconut milk kefir

1 tablespoon cider vinegar

¹/₃ cup canola oil

1 cup raisins

1. Preheat the oven to 325°F and lightly grease a 9 x 5-inch loaf pan.

2. In a large mixing bowl, whisk together the rice flour, potato starch, sorghum flour, xanthan gum, salt, baking powder, baking soda, and sugar.

3. In another bowl, whisk together the applesauce, coconut milk kefir, cider vinegar, and canola oil. Pour the wet ingredients into the dry ingredients and stir together until the dry ingredients are just moistened. The batter will be lumpy, but there should be no remaining dry patches.

4. Fold in the raisins and pour the batter into the prepared loaf pan. Bake the bread for 70 minutes or until a wooden skewer inserted in the center comes out clean.

5. Cool the bread in the pan for 15 minutes and then turn the loaf out onto a wire cooling rack to cool completely.

6. Leftovers may be stored in an airtight container, refrigerated, for up to 3 days. The completely cooled loaf may also be frozen in an airtight container for up to 3 months.

Stuffing Cornbread

Thanksgiving can be a tough holiday for those of us with food allergies, because so many foods that we consider typically American are loaded with some combination of gluten, dairy, soy, nuts, and eggs. Traditional stuffing, even the cornbread variety, is usually made with wheat, often bound with lots of egg. Thus, I had not had stuffing in years until I developed this recipe. What I love about this recipe is that it is actually a two for one, because you are getting your Thanksgiving stuffing and the cornbread side all in one dish! It is simply cornbread seasoned with all the stuffing herbs and some bacon. Savory yet sweet, sage-y, and moist, it is the perfect accompaniment to a Thanksgiving turkey roasted golden brown. This cornbread must be baked in a pan, however. Do not try stuffing a turkey with it or it will not work. SERVES 12

1. Preheat the oven to 425°F and grease a 9 x 13-inch pan or a 13-inch paella pan with canola oil. Set the pan aside.

2. In a skillet cook the bacon over medium-high heat until it is crispy. Remove the bacon to paper towels to drain, reserving the pan drippings. When it is cool enough to handle, crumble or chop the bacon and set aside.

3. Sauté the celery and onion in the bacon grease until the onion is translucent and the celery has softened. Stir in the salt and pepper. Remove the pan from the heat, stir in the poultry seasoning, and let the vegetables cool slightly while you prepare the cornbread batter.

4. In a large bowl, thoroughly whisk together the cornmeal, Chinese rice flour, potato starch, sorghum flour, sugar, baking powder, baking soda, and xanthan gum. Pour in the canola oil, applesauce, and chicken stock.

5. Stir the cider vinegar into the water and add it to the batter. Stir the batter until the ingredients are thoroughly incorporated and no dry bits remain. Fold in the bacon, sautéed vegetables, and golden raisins.

6. Pour the batter into the prepared pan, smooth the top with a knife, and bake for 22 minutes or until the top is golden and a toothpick inserted in the center comes out clean.

7. Remove the cornbread from the oven, let it cool slightly, and serve warm. Although the cornbread is best eaten immediately, leftovers may be stored in an airtight container for up to 3 days.

4 slices soy-free bacon
2 ribs celery, chopped
1 small onion, chopped
1/2 teaspoon salt
Dash pepper
1 tablespoon poultry seasoning
2 cups cornmeal
1 1/3 cups Chinese rice flour or superfine rice flour
1/2 cup potato starch
1/4 cup sorghum flour
1/2 cup sugar
3 teaspoons baking powder
1 teaspoon baking soda
1 1/4 teaspoons xanthan gum
1/2 cup canola oil
2 tablespoons unsweetened applesauce
1 cup chicken stock (page 112)
2 tablespoons cider vinegar
1 cup water
2/3 cup golden raisins

Potato Latkes

At our house I often struggle with making things that our entire family will eat. Inevitably my children ask me first thing in the morning what we are having for dinner, and I know that when I say latkes, I will receive a cheer rather than a groan. Needless to say, I make these frequently. SERVES 4

1 pound potatoes (about 2 large baking potatoes), peeled and shredded
2 teaspoons potato starch
½ teaspoon salt
Dash pepper
3 tablespoons canola oil
Applesauce for serving (optional)

1. In a large bowl, combine the shredded potatoes, potato starch, salt, and pepper.

2. Heat the canola oil in a large skillet over medium-high heat.

3. Using your hands, form ¼-cup scoops of potato mixture into patties, squeezing out the excess moisture as you form them; there will be a lot of excess moisture.

4. Place the patties in the hot oil and fry for 4 minutes. After 4 minutes, flip the latkes, pressing down on the patties with the spatula to ensure that the patties remain intact. Fry for an additional 4 minutes.

5. Remove the latkes from the heat and serve them immediately with applesauce, if desired.

6. The latkes are best eaten immediately, but completely cooled leftovers may be frozen with squares of wax paper between them for up to 3 months and then reheated in the oven at 450°F for 15 minutes.

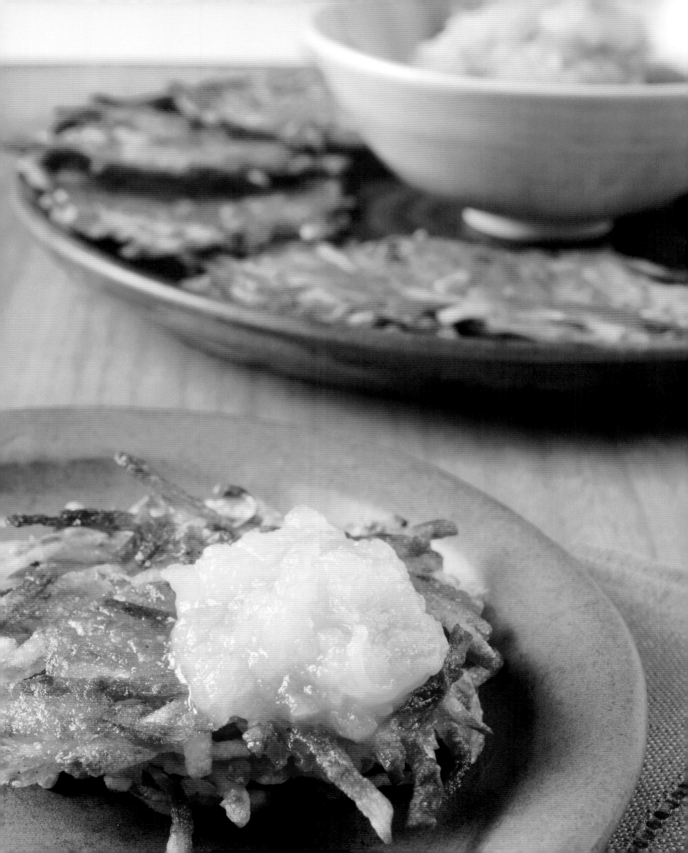

Onion Rings

I think the hardest thing to give up—other than a lot of desserts—after I found out I had food allergies was fried food. I know it isn't good for me, but I can't be healthy all the time! Anyway, the fryer oil in restaurants is used for all the fried food they serve, so thanks to mozzarella sticks and chicken tenders and whatever else the restaurant cooks in there, french fries and everything else gets contaminated with wheat. I bake my own fries now. However, it wasn't until I was writing this book that I started playing around with things like onion rings. Of course the breading always made this favorite off-limits, but I found a way around it. My All-Purpose Breading (see page 66) combined with some rice milk and vinegar is the perfect stand-in for the traditional batter and egg. One bite and I was transported back to the Spot, an authentic 1950s drive-in in my hometown that up until about ten years ago served their food on a tray attached to the window of your car.

SERVES 4

Canola oil for frying
1 cup plain rice milk
1 tablespoon cider vinegar
1¼ cups All-Purpose Breading
   (see page 66)
1 large onion, cut into ¼-inch
   slices

1. Pour the canola oil into a fryer according to the fryer directions. If you are not using a fryer, pour 4 to 5 inches of canola oil into a large heavy skillet. Preheat the fryer or the oil in the pan to 350°F.

2. Pour the rice milk into a large shallow bowl and stir in the cider vinegar.

3. Pour the All-Purpose Breading into another large shallow bowl.

4. Working with one or two slices at a time, dip the onion in the rice milk mixture and then in the All-Purpose Breading. Repeat the process and then place the double-coated onion rings in the preheated oil.

5. Fry the onion rings for 3 minutes or until they are golden brown, turning if necessary. Continue double-coating the remaining onion rings and frying them a few at a time so as not to overcrowd the fryer until all of the onion rings have been fried.

6. Drain the onion rings on a paper towel–lined plate and serve immediately.

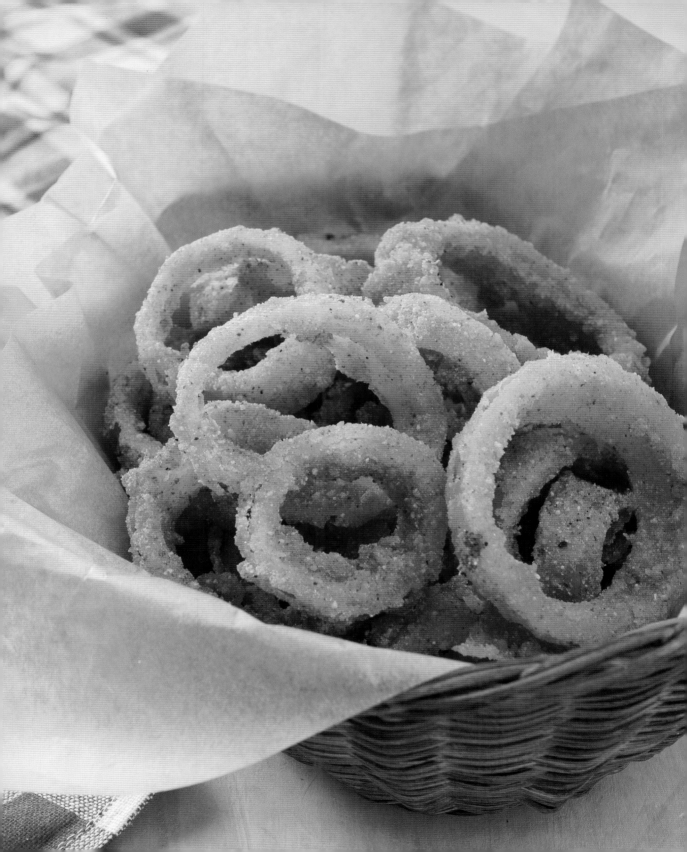

Basic Chocolate Wafers

Mint Thin Wafers

Animal Crackers

Golden Sponge Cakes
with Cream Filling

Whoopie Pies

Supermarket Frosting

Chocolate Ganache Frosting

S'Mores Cookies

Double Chocolate Chip
Ice Cream

Vanilla Pudding

Basic Double Piecrust

Cherry Pie

Pumpkin Pie Bars
with Oatmeal Raisin Crust

Pretend Peanut Butter Kisses

Chocolate Chip Cookies

Gingerbread Men with
Lemon Icing

Texas Sheet Cake

Cream-Filled Oatmeal Cookie
Sandwiches

Sweet Potato Pie

Not Really Peanut Butter Fudge

Chocolate Egg Cream

Snickerdoodles

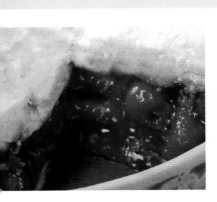 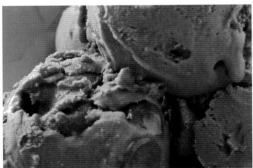 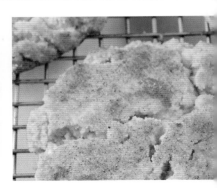

Desserts

Dessert will always be my favorite course, so much so that I frequently opt to eat it first! When you have food allergies and so much is off-limits, it is often too hard to wait until the end of the meal to enjoy something that is not only sweet and delicious, but also gluten, dairy, soy, nut, and egg free. There are so many desserts that I most closely associate with comfort food I missed, so I wrote the following recipes to revisit those childhood classics in a safe way. From Thin Mints™ to animal crackers to Twinkies™, they are all celebrated here, and so are many others that you may have missed, too.

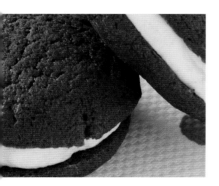
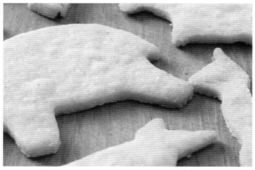
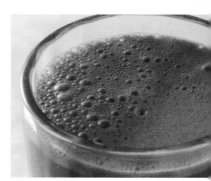

Basic Chocolate Wafers

Sometimes a recipe is so versatile that it works in several different recipes. Use these Basic Chocolate Wafers in my Mint Thin Wafers (see page 147), cut them in fun shapes and bake them dusted with sanding sugar, or put a spoonful of Supermarket Frosting (see page 154) between two for an allergy-free chocolate sandwich cookie. Whichever way you choose to use them, they are the perfect crunchy texture with a rich chocolate flavor. MAKES 48 3½-INCH CUTOUTS

1½ cups Chinese or superfine rice flour
⅔ cup potato starch
¼ cup sorghum flour
⅓ cup unsweetened cocoa powder
¾ teaspoon baking powder
¼ teaspoon salt
2 teaspoons powdered vanilla rice milk
1 teaspoon xanthan gum
1 cup leaf lard
1 cup sugar
¼ cup applesauce
1 teaspoon vanilla extract
3 tablespoons plus 1 teaspoon water

1. Preheat the oven to 350°F. Line two baking sheets with parchment paper and set them aside until you are ready to use them.

2. In a large mixing bowl, whisk together the rice flour, potato starch, sorghum flour, unsweetened cocoa powder, baking powder, salt, powdered vanilla rice milk, and xanthan gum; set aside.

3. In the bowl of a stand mixer, cream together the leaf lard and sugar until they are light and fluffy. Beat in the applesauce and vanilla extract. Scrape down the sides.

4. Add in the dry ingredients, alternating with the water and stir until the dough comes together.

5. Using your hands, pull the dough into a ball. Split the ball in two and wrap half of it in plastic and store it in the refrigerator until you are ready to roll it out. Place the unwrapped ball of dough between two sheets of parchment paper and roll it out to ¼-inch thickness. Cut the dough with a 3⅓-inch round cutter. Repeat until you have used both balls of dough.

6. Place the cut cookies on the prepared baking sheets and bake in the preheated oven for 11 minutes or until golden at the edges.

7. Let the cookies cool on the sheets for 5 minutes and then remove them to a wire rack to cool completely. Leftover cookies may be stored in an airtight container for up to 5 days.

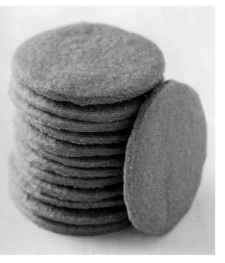

Mint Thin Wafers

I joined the Brownies in second grade because I wanted the uniform. It's true. I loved the necktie and the tunic over the pants. I dropped out after I got it, but not before my mother became the "cookie chairwoman" and ran the cookie campaign out of our garage. When March rolled around the year I was diagnosed with food allergies, I was disappointed that I couldn't indulge in my beloved Thin Mints™. Disappointment be darned. MAKES ABOUT 48 COOKIES

1. Preheat the oven to 350°F. Line two baking sheets with parchment paper; set aside.

2. Make the Basic Chocolate Wafers according to the recipe directions.

3. When the cookies are completely cooled, melt the chocolate chips with the peppermint extract in the top of a double boiler set to simmer. When the chocolate is two-thirds of the way melted, remove it from the heat and stir it until it is completely smooth. Let the chocolate cool slightly.

4. Set a cooling rack over a sheet of parchment paper. When the chocolate has cooled slightly, about 5 to 10 minutes, take one cookie at a time and lower it into the melted chocolate, covering the entire cookie with chocolate. Remove the covered cookie to the cooling rack to cool and let the chocolate set.

5. Completely cooled and set cookies may be stored, refrigerated, in an airtight container for up to 3 days. I recommend placing wax paper between the cookies if you will be stacking them for storage. These cookies may also be frozen with wax paper between them, in an airtight container, for up to 3 months.

1 recipe Basic Chocolate
  Wafers (see page 146)
1 pound gluten-, dairy-,
  soy-, nut-, and egg-free
  semisweet chocolate chips
1 teaspoon peppermint extract

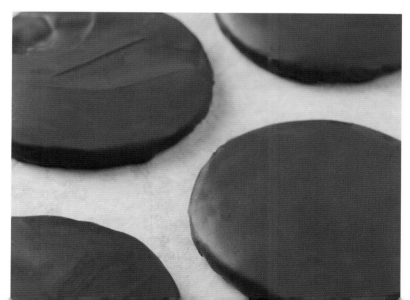

Animal Crackers

One of my daughters' favorite songs is Shirley Temple's "Animal Crackers in My Soup." They make me listen to it on repeat every time we are in the car. So, of course, I had to make these little cookies for them. MAKES ABOUT 100 CRACKERS

2 teaspoons powdered vanilla rice milk

2 cups Chinese or superfine rice flour

$^2/_3$ cup potato starch

$^1/_3$ cup sorghum flour

1 teaspoon baking powder

$^1/_4$ teaspoon nutmeg

1 teaspoon mace

$^1/_2$ teaspoon salt

1 teaspoon xanthan gum

$^3/_4$ cup plus 3 tablespoons leaf lard

1 cup plus 1 tablespoon granulated sugar

$^1/_4$ cup applesauce

1 teaspoon vanilla extract

2 tablespoons water

White sanding sugar for dusting (optional)

1. Preheat the oven to 350°F. Line two baking sheets with parchment paper and set them aside until ready to use.

2. In a large bowl whisk together the powdered vanilla rice milk, Chinese rice flour, potato starch, sorghum flour, baking powder, nutmeg, mace, salt, and xanthan gum; set aside.

3. In the bowl of a stand mixer, cream together the leaf lard and granulated sugar until they are light and fluffy. Beat in the applesauce and vanilla extract and scrape down the sides.

4. Stir in the dry ingredients. Once the mixture begins to look coarse and crumbly, stir in the 2 tablespoons of water and then beat the dough on medium speed until it comes together. Remove the bowl from the mixer and, using your hands, gather the dough into a ball.

5. Split the dough in half and place half on a sheet of parchment paper. Tightly wrap the other half in plastic wrap and set it aside until ready to use. Roll out the first half between two sheets of parchment paper to $^1/_4$-inch thickness. Using animal-shaped cutters, cut the dough into cookies. Continue rerolling and cutting the dough until you have used it all.

6. Place the cut cookies on the prepared baking sheets, dust with the sanding sugar, if using, and bake for 11 minutes or until the edges are just golden.

7. Remove the cookies to cooling racks to cool completely before serving.

8. Store the finished cookies in an airtight container at room temperature for 3 to 5 days or freeze them for up to 3 months.

Note: Williams-Sonoma makes an adorable set of animal cracker cutters, but mini animal cutters work fine, too.

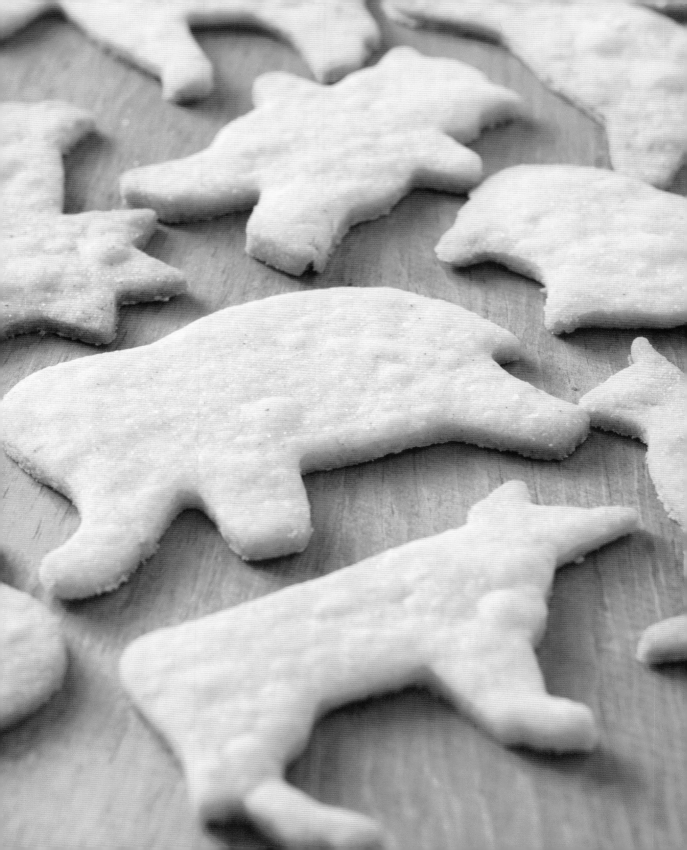

Golden Sponge Cakes with Cream Filling

Without fail my brother and I always fought over the last Twinkie™. I loved them and usually whined to my mother until my brother had no choice but to hand over the last of our stash. Now I can make as many as I want, whenever I want, and I don't have to worry about allergic reactions. I use an éclair pan for this recipe to get the perfect shape. These pans are easy to find in most large housewares stores or online at Amazon. SERVES 12

1. Preheat the oven to 350°F. Lightly grease 12 éclair molds with canola oil and set them aside.

2. In a large bowl whisk together the Chinese rice flour, potato starch, sorghum flour, xanthan gum, baking soda, baking powder, salt, and powdered vanilla rice milk.

3. In a small bowl mix together the water and the cider vinegar; set aside.

4. In the bowl of a stand mixer, cream together the organic palm fruit oil shortening and sugar until they are light and fluffy. Beat in the applesauce and then stir in the dry ingredients in 3 additions, beginning and ending with the dry ingredients and alternating with the water and cider vinegar mixture.

5. Pour the batter into the prepared éclair pans and bake for 18 to 20 minutes or until a toothpick inserted in the center comes out clean.

6. Remove the éclair pan from the oven and allow the cakes to cool completely in the pan before removing to a cooling rack.

7. When the cakes have cooled completely, load a pastry bag, fitted with a #4 tip, with Supermarket Frosting. Insert the tip about 1/4 inch from one end of the cake halfway into the flat side of the cake and fill with frosting, being careful not to overfill or the cake will break. Repeat in the center of the cake and then one more time 1/4 inch from the end of the cake.

8. Store in an airtight container in the refrigerator or at room temperature for up to 3 days.

2 cups Chinese rice flour
2/3 cup potato starch
1/3 cup sorghum flour
1 teaspoon xanthan gum
1 teaspoon baking soda
3 teaspoons baking powder
1 teaspoon salt
1 tablespoon powdered vanilla rice milk
1 cup water
1 tablespoon cider vinegar
1 cup organic palm fruit oil shortening
2 cups granulated sugar
1/2 cup unsweetened applesauce
1 recipe Supermarket Frosting (see page 154)

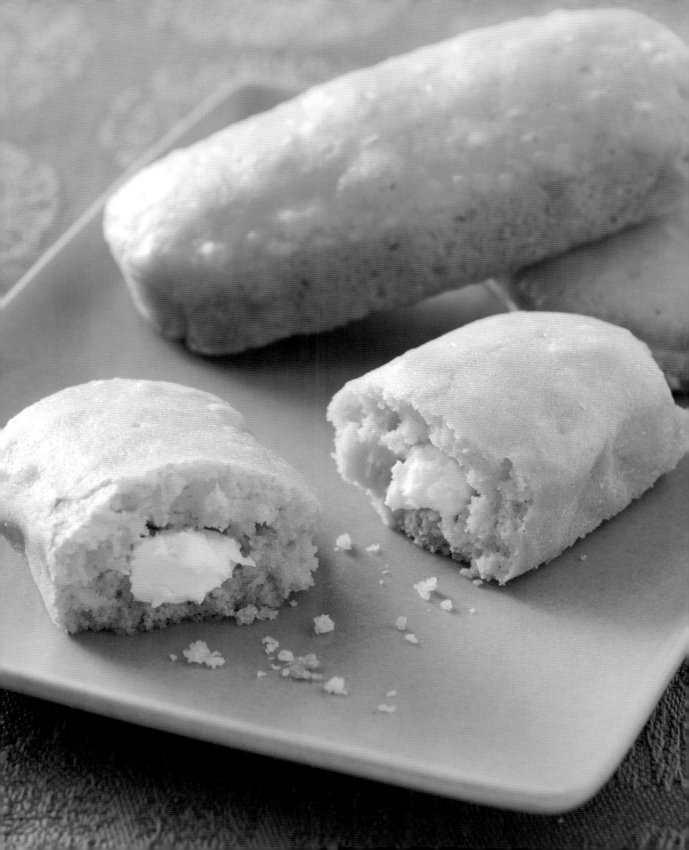

Whoopie Pies

I had never even heard of whoopie pies until I moved to New York City. They are actually a Maine tradition, not a New York City thing, but when I first arrived here, they were starting to gain popularity and could be found in a lot of the high-end food stores like Zabar's and Citarella. It's funny that they are considered a fancy treat here, since I have been told that whoopie pies are available for purchase in most gas stations in Maine. Once I tasted them, I became a whoopie pie devotee. They really are the perfect dessert because they are cake accompanied by an abnormally large helping of frosting, which is just the way that I like cake. Eager to continue eating whoopie pies after I found out I was allergic to wheat and eggs, I made sure that I developed a gluten-, dairy-, soy-, nut-, and egg-free version. Chocolaty, creamy, and cakey, I think that you will agree that this dessert truly is a classic. MAKES 13 WHOOPIE PIES

1⅓ cups Chinese rice flour
½ cup potato starch
¼ cup sorghum flour
¼ cup unsweetened cocoa powder
1 teaspoon baking soda
1 teaspoon baking powder
1 teaspoon xanthan gum
1 teaspoon salt
1 tablespoon powdered vanilla rice milk
1 cup water
1 tablespoon cider vinegar
½ cup organic palm fruit oil shortening
1 cup dark brown sugar
2 tablespoons unsweetened applesauce
1 recipe Supermarket Frosting (see page 154)

1. Preheat the oven to 350°F. Line two baking sheets with parchment paper and set them aside.

2. In a large bowl whisk together the Chinese rice flour, potato starch, sorghum flour, cocoa powder, baking soda, baking powder, xanthan gum, salt, and powdered vanilla rice milk; set aside.

3. In a small bowl combine the water and cider vinegar. Set aside.

4. In the bowl of a stand mixer, cream the organic palm fruit oil shortening and dark brown sugar until fluffy. Beat in the applesauce and scrape down the sides. Add the dry ingredients alternately with the water and cider vinegar combination, starting and ending with the dry ingredients. Blend until smooth.

5. Using a small ice cream scoop, release the batter onto the prepared sheets. Bake for 10 to 12 minutes or until the cakes are firm to the touch and a toothpick inserted in the center comes out clean. Remove the finished cakes to cooling racks to cool completely.

6. When the cakes are completely cooled, frost the flat side with Supermarket Frosting and then place another cake on top to form a soft sandwich cookie.

7. Eat the whoopie pies immediately or store them, refrigerated, in an airtight container for 3 days.

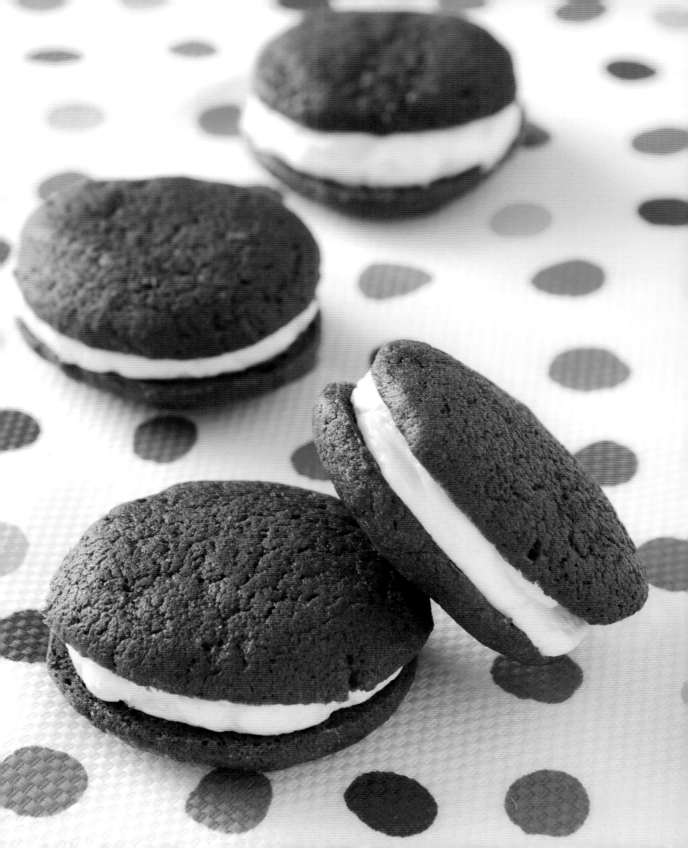

Supermarket Frosting

Growing up I loved the huge, brightly colored roses on the birthday cakes from the supermarket. As my mother always made our birthday cakes, it was a rare treat (and one usually reserved for school birthday parties) that I got to eat that yummy frosting. This tastes just like it, only it is gluten, dairy, soy, nut, egg and trans-fat free. MAKES 3 CUPS

³/₄ cup organic palm fruit oil shortening
¹/₃ cup powdered vanilla rice milk
5 cups confectioners' sugar, sifted
¹/₄ cup plus 1 tablespoon water
¹/₂ teaspoon salt
1 teaspoon vanilla extract

1. In the bowl of a stand mixer, cream the organic palm fruit oil shortening and the powdered vanilla rice milk until they are light and fluffy.

2. Stir in the confectioners' sugar 1 cup at a time. The mixture will be crumbly.

3. Slowly stir in the water, salt, and vanilla extract and then beat the frosting for 3 minutes on medium high.

4. Use the frosting immediately or store it in an airtight container with plastic wrap pressed directly on top of it in the refrigerator for 3 to 5 days or, in the freezer for up to 3 months. Thaw the frosting completely and beat it again before using.

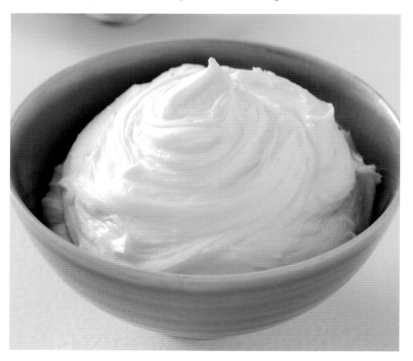

Chocolate Ganache Frosting

This frosting reminds me of that superthick, rich frosting you can buy in a can in the supermarket. I used to eat it by the spoonful, but then I found out that a lot of the canned brands contain wheat. I also closely read the ingredients list and found that most of the canned varieties don't contain any real food, so I got to work to create a healthier replacement. This is as rich as ganache but as smooth, fluffy, and creamy as a traditional chocolate frosting. MAKES 1½ CUPS

1. Place the chocolate chips, Lyle's Golden Syrup or corn syrup, coconut milk, and espresso crystals in a small saucepan. Stirring constantly, so as not to scorch the chocolate, melt the mixture over low heat.

2. When the chocolate is two-thirds of the way melted, remove from the heat and continue stirring until it is completely smooth. When the ganache is completely smooth, beat in the confectioners' sugar and canola oil with a hand mixer until a thick, smooth frosting has formed.

3. Leftovers may be stored, refrigerated, for up to 5 days. Let the frosting stand at room temperature until it is soft enough to spread.

10 ounces gluten-, dairy-, soy-, nut-, and egg-free semisweet chocolate chips
1 tablespoon Lyle's Golden Syrup or corn syrup
⅓ cup well-shaken canned coconut milk
¼ teaspoon espresso crystals
1 cup sifted confectioners' sugar
1 tablespoon canola oil

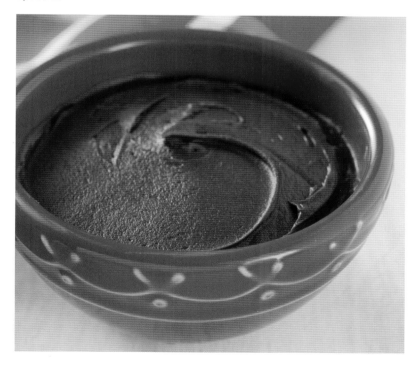

S'Mores Cookies

To me no dessert says summer like a s'more. On summer weekends we inevitably end up on the beach with friends, and these trips are usually followed by a really great potluck dinner, rounded out by a bonfire and s'mores. No matter how often it happens, the children squeal with glee when we announce dessert. I love s'mores but can't eat the graham crackers, so I set out to create an allergy-free version for myself. I can't wait for summer to eat these on the beach! MAKES 20 S'MORES COOKIES

1½ cups superfine or Chinese rice flour

½ cup potato starch

¼ cup sorghum flour

1 teaspoon baking soda

1 teaspoon baking powder

1 teaspoon xanthan gum

1 teaspoon salt

¾ teaspoon cinnamon

1 cup organic palm fruit oil shortening

1¼ cups light brown sugar

¼ cup honey

2 tablespoons ground flaxseed meal

6 tablespoons water

1 3.5-ounce gluten-, dairy-, soy-, nut-, and egg-free 85% cacao chocolate bar, broken into 20 squares (see Where to Shop Guide)

20 large marshmallows

1. Preheat the oven to 350°F and line two baking sheets with parchment paper.

2. Whisk together the rice flour, potato starch, sorghum flour, baking soda, baking powder, xanthan gum, salt, and cinnamon in a large mixing bowl.

3. In the bowl of a stand mixer, cream together the organic palm fruit oil shortening and brown sugar until they are fluffy. Scrape down the sides and beat in the honey.

4. Mix together the flaxseed meal and the water and add this mixture to the batter. Beat the batter until it is light and fluffy again. Scrape down the sides.

5. Slowly stir in the dry ingredients and mix until the dough comes together and all the ingredients are evenly incorporated.

6. With a 1½-inch-diameter ice cream scoop, scoop the batter out onto the prepared sheets to form 20 cookies. Top each cookie with a square of chocolate.

7. Bake the cookies for 11 minutes or until the edges are just golden. Remove the cookies from the oven and top each with a marshmallow. Turn on the broiler and place the cookies under the broiler for 30 seconds or until the marshmallows are just golden. Watch the marshmallows carefully, as they can burn in a flash.

8. Let the cookies cool on the cookie sheets for 10 minutes and then remove them to cooling racks to cool completely. Store the cookies in an airtight container at room temperature for up to 3 days.

Note: If you are having trouble finding allergy-appropriate chocolate bars, press 1 teaspoon of gluten-, dairy-, soy-, nut-, and egg-free chocolate chips into the top of the cookie before baking.

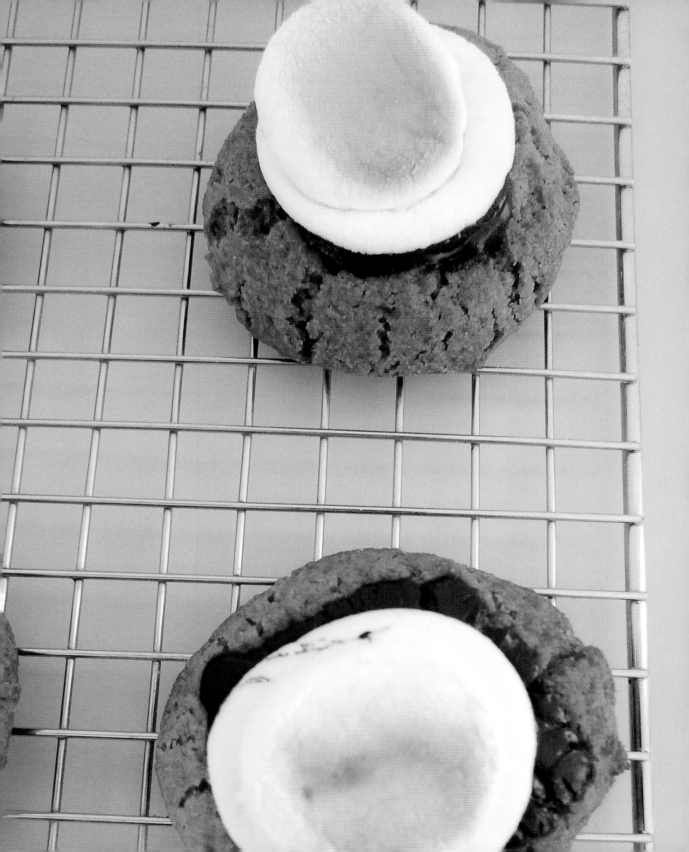

Double Chocolate Chip Ice Cream

In my opinion summer is not summer without ice cream, and ice cream is not ice cream if it is not chocolate. The problem is that for those of us with food allergies, many brands of ice cream are off-limits. Obviously most ice cream is made with dairy, but not everyone knows that many premium ice creams also contain eggs. I love to make my own ice cream because I can't tolerate eggs, and last year I began playing around with a dairy-free, homemade ice cream alternative. I think you will be amazed by the creaminess and the intensity of the chocolate in this recipe. Just make sure you have a really good scoop—as you may already know from commercial brands, coconut milk ice cream can get very hard after it has been frozen for several hours. SERVES 8

¼ cup sugar

3 tablespoons cornstarch

3 cups canned coconut milk (not lite), well shaken, divided

1½ cups dairy- and soy-free chocolate chips, divided

1. In a large bowl whisk together the sugar and cornstarch; set aside.

2. Pour 2¾ cups of the coconut milk and 1 cup of the chocolate chips into a medium saucepan and bring to a boil over medium heat, stirring constantly.

3. Just before the coconut milk begins to boil, whisk the remaining coconut milk into the cornstarch mixture until it is smooth.

4. When the coconut milk boils, pour in the cornstarch mixture and cook, boiling gently and whisking constantly, for 3 minutes. The mixture will become very thick.

5. After 3 minutes, remove the mixture from the heat and let it cool completely at room temperature for about 1½ hours; do not refrigerate.

6. When the mixture has cooled completely, pour it into an ice-cream machine and process according to the machine instructions. Five minutes before the end of the cycle, pour in the remaining ½ cup of the chocolate chips. When the machine reaches the end of its cycle, remove the mixture to a plastic airtight container and freeze for 2 hours.

7. Using an ice-cream scooper dipped in hot water, scoop and serve. Store, frozen in an airtight container, for up to 3 months.

Note: If the ice cream is too hard to scoop, which is a hazard with coconut milk, microwave the container in 5 to 7 second increments until the ice cream is just scoopable.

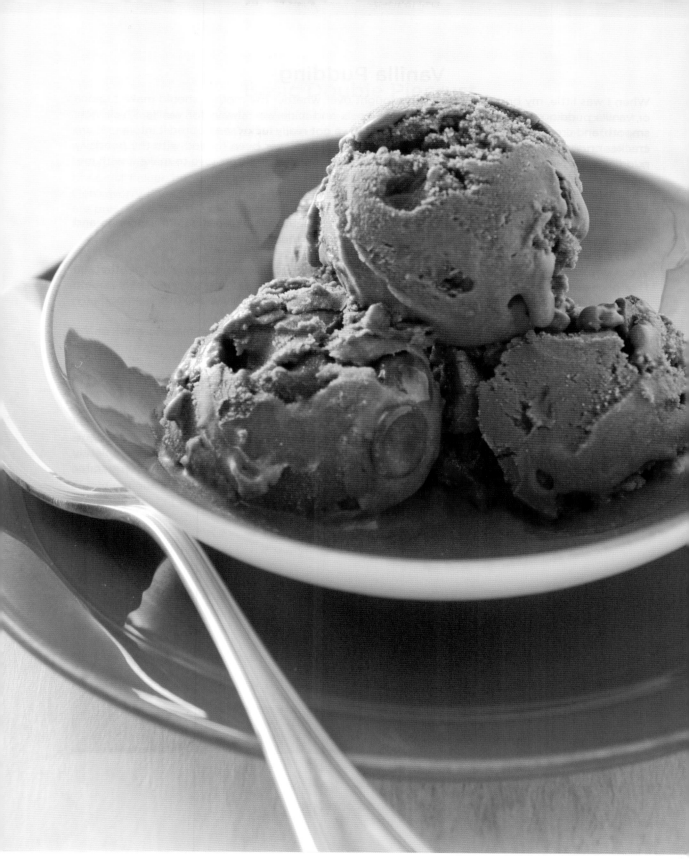

Cherry Pie

This is a pie I associate with early June on my parents' screened-in porch. Pies are all the rage these days, with pie bakeries popping up everywhere. A master pie baker, my mother was really ahead of the curve. When I learned that I had food allergies, I did not worry too much about pie, because I figured I would just forego the crust and eat generous helpings of the filling. As someone who prefers to make cakes, I wasn't aware that many pie fillings contain flour, too. This pie recipe uses cornstarch to thicken the filling, keeping it gluten-free. If cornstarch doesn't work for you or your allergies, feel free to substitute tapioca starch. SERVES 8-10

1 Basic Double Piecrust (see page 161)
2 pounds pitted cherries, halved
1 cup sugar
1/8 teaspoon salt
3 tablespoons cornstarch
Canola oil for brushing
2 teaspoons granulated sugar

1. Preheat the oven to 400°F. Prepare the Basic Double Piecrust according to the recipe and set it aside.

2. In a large mixing bowl, combine the cherries, sugar, salt, and cornstarch. Pour the cherry mixture into the prepared crust, top with the second half of the crust, and crimp the edges. Cut 4 small slits in the top to allow steam to escape. Spray or lightly brush the top crust with a little canola oil. Sprinkle the pie with the 2 tea-spoons of granulated sugar.

3. Bake the pie for 50 minutes or until the cherry filling is bubbly and the edges of the piecrust have begun to turn golden.

4. Cool the pie completely before serving it. Store any uneaten pie, covered and refrigerated, for up to 3 days.

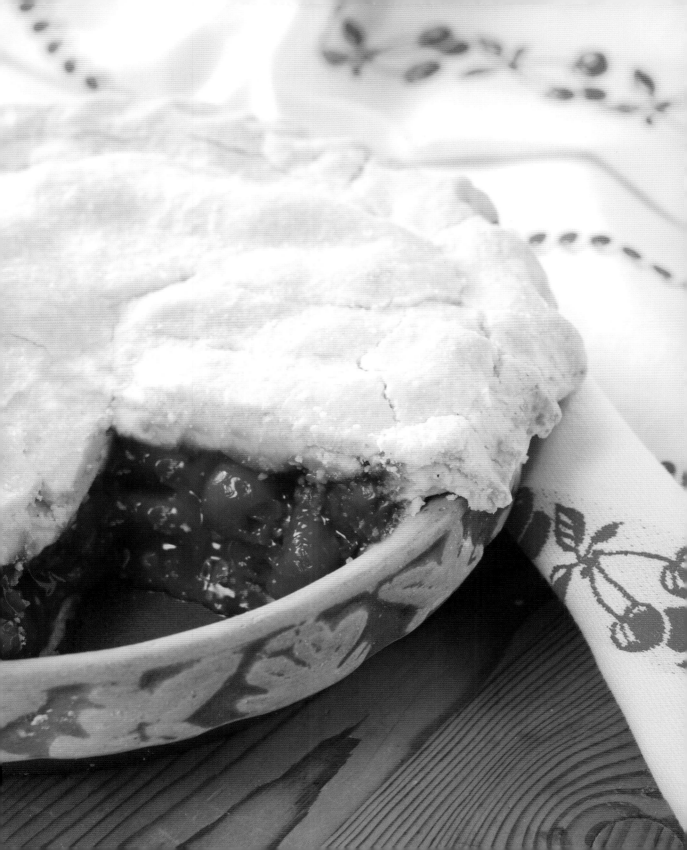

Pumpkin Pie Bars with Oatmeal Raisin Crust

When I was pregnant with my first daughter, before I was diagnosed with food allergies, my husband and I used to go to a little cafe once a week to feed my cravings for sweets. One week we stumbled upon a version of these pumpkin squares, and I was instantly hooked. I finally got around to making an allergy-free recipe that is a nearly exact replica of the original. Serve these with your favorite allergy-friendly whipped topping or ice cream for a special treat. MAKES 24 BARS

Oatmeal Raisin Crust

1 cup Chinese or superfine rice flour
1/3 cup potato starch
3 tablespoons sorghum flour
1 teaspoon baking soda
1 teaspoon baking powder
1 teaspoon cinnamon
1 teaspoon xanthan gum
1 1/3 cups organic palm oil shortening
1 cup brown sugar
1/4 cup granulated sugar
1/2 cup applesauce
1 teaspoon vanilla extract
3 cups certified gluten-free oats
1 cup raisins

Filling

2 cups pumpkin puree
2/3 cup light brown sugar
1/3 cup maple syrup
1/2 teaspoon salt
1 tablespoon pumpkin pie spice
Pinch ground black pepper
1 tablespoon bourbon (optional)
1 teaspoon vanilla extract (omit if using French vanilla creamer, below)
1 cup French vanilla or plain So Delicious coconut milk creamer
1/4 cup plus 2 teaspoons cornstarch

1. Preheat the oven to 350°F and lightly grease a 9 x 13-inch pan with a little organic palm oil shortening. Set the pan aside until ready to use.

2. In a large bowl whisk together the rice flour, potato starch, sorghum flour, baking soda, baking powder, cinnamon, and xanthan gum; set aside.

3. In the bowl of a stand mixer, cream together the shortening and sugars until they are light and fluffy. Beat in the applesauce and vanilla extract and scrape down the sides.

4. Slowly mix in the flour mixture until it is completely combined and then scrape down the sides again. Fold in the oats and then the raisins.

5. Spread the batter in the bottom of the prepared pan and bake in the preheated oven for 8 minutes.

6. While the crust is baking, prepare the filling. In a large mixing bowl, place the pumpkin; brown sugar; maple syrup; salt; pumpkin pie spice; pepper; bourbon, if using; and vanilla extract, if using. Stir the mixture until it is thoroughly combined.

7. In a small bowl add 1/4 cup of the coconut milk creamer to the cornstarch and stir until the mixture is smooth. Add the remaining coconut milk creamer and stir again. Pour the cornstarch and creamer mix into the pumpkin mix and stir until it is completely incorporated. Pour the custard mixture onto the cookie crust and return the pan to the oven for 55 to 60 minutes or until the custard is set.

8. Remove the bars from the oven and cool completely before cutting them. Serve immediately or store leftovers in an airtight container, refrigerated, for up to 3 days.

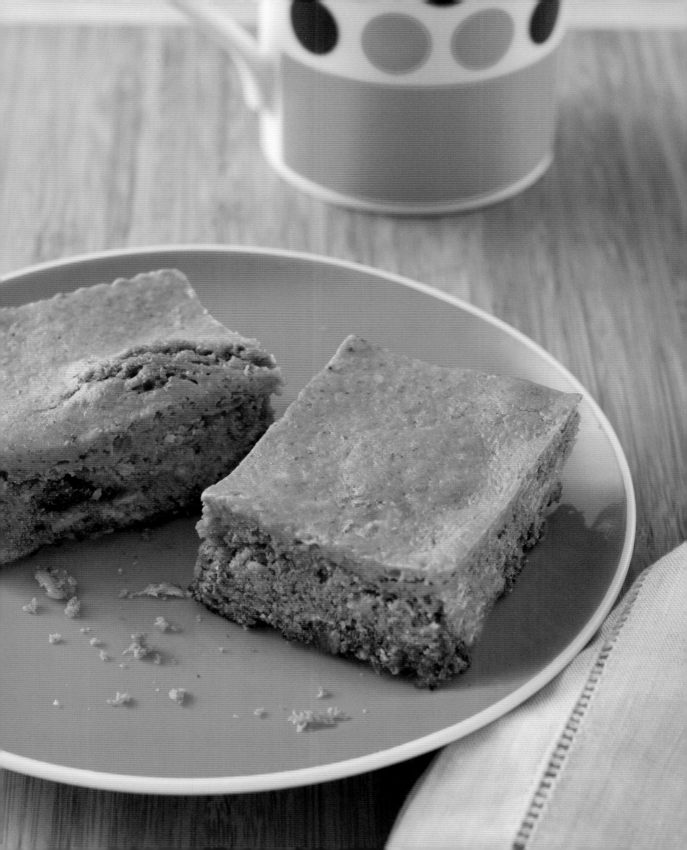

Pretend Peanut Butter Kisses

Remember when you were little and other kids' moms sent in cookies for birthday celebrations? Well, where I grew up, these were often a favorite for such occasions. Unfortunately today peanut butter is forbidden in many classrooms, and chocolate kisses contain dairy and soy. Never fear, here is an allergy-friendly stand-in. These are great for the holidays, at bake sales, and, of course, at school birthday parties. MAKES ABOUT 55 COOKIES

1 cup plus 2 tablespoons
   superfine rice flour
²/₃ cup potato starch
2 tablespoons plus 1 teaspoon
   sorghum flour
³/₄ teaspoon xanthan gum
1 teaspoon baking powder
¹/₈ teaspoon baking soda
¹/₂ cup organic palm fruit oil
   shortening
¹/₂ cup sunflower seed butter
¹/₂ cup granulated sugar
¹/₂ cup light brown sugar
¹/₄ cup applesauce
2 tablespoons water
¹/₄ cup granulated sugar
1 recipe Chocolate Ganache
   Frosting (see page 155)

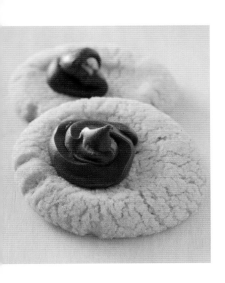

1. Preheat the oven to 350°F. Line two baking sheets with parchment paper; set aside.

2. In a large mixing bowl, whisk together the rice flour, potato starch, sorghum flour, xanthan gum, baking powder, and baking soda.

3. In the bowl of a stand mixer, cream the palm fruit oil shortening, sunflower seed butter, the ¹/₂ cup of granulated sugar, and the brown sugar until they are light and fluffy. Scrape down the sides of the bowl.

4. Add the applesauce and water and beat until both are combined. Scrape down the sides again.

5. Slowly add the dry ingredients, stirring the batter until all of the dry ingredients are incorporated.

6. Pour the ¹/₄ cup of granulated sugar into a shallow bowl. With a tablespoon measure, scoop the dough and roll it between your hands to form 1-inch balls. Roll each ball in the sugar and place it on the cookie sheet about 1 inch apart. Using the knuckle of your bent forefinger, place an indentation in the center of each ball. Bake for 12 minutes or until the edges are just lightly browned.

7. Remove the cookies from the oven and let them cool for 5 minutes on the cookie sheets before removing them to cooling racks to cool completely.

8. When the cookies are cool, load a pastry bag fitted with a #4 tip with Chocolate Ganache Frosting. Fill each indentation with a dollop of ganache.

9. Store uneaten cookies in an airtight container, refrigerated, for 3 to 5 days.

Chocolate Chip Cookies

Whenever I've been abroad and told people that I love to bake, the first thing they ask is whether or not I'll whip up a batch of chocolate chip cookies. Who doesn't have a fond memory of chocolate chips? These cookies are not my original Betsy & Claude Baking Co. recipe, but they are a nod to the exceedingly popular Tate's cookies that have swept New York City. These are thin, crisp, and lacy with a great flavor. They are delicious made into chipwiches with a scoop of dairy-free vanilla ice cream sandwiched between two of the cookies. **MAKES 36 COOKIES**

1. Preheat the oven to 350°F. Line two baking sheets with parchment paper and set aside.

2. In a small bowl combine the flaxseed meal and water; set aside.

3. In a large bowl whisk together the Chinese rice flour, potato starch, sorghum flour, baking soda, baking power, salt, and xanthan gum; set aside.

4. In the bowl of a stand mixer, cream the shortening and sugars until they are very light and fluffy. Scrape down the sides of the bowl.

5. Add the flaxseed meal mixture and vanilla extract. Beat the batter until it is light and fluffy again and then scrape down the sides.

6. Stir in the dry ingredients until they are thoroughly combined, and then fold in the chocolate chips.

7. Using a 1½-inch-diameter ice cream scoop, scoop the batter onto the prepared baking sheets. Bake the cookies in the preheated oven for 15 minutes. Cool on the baking sheets for 15 minutes and then move to cooling racks to cool completely.

8. The cookies may be stored in an airtight container at room temperature for 3 to 5 days or frozen in an airtight container for up to 3 months.

2 tablespoons ground flaxseed meal
6 tablespoons water
1⅓ cups Chinese rice flour
½ cup potato starch
¼ cup sorghum flour
1 teaspoon baking soda
1 teaspoon baking powder
1 teaspoon salt
⅜ teaspoon xanthan gum
1 cup organic palm fruit oil shortening
1 cup white sugar
¾ cup dark brown sugar
1½ teaspoons vanilla extract
2 cups gluten-, dairy-, soy-, nut-, and egg-free chocolate chips

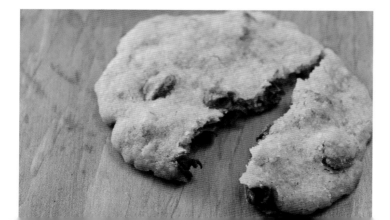

Gingerbread Men with Lemon Icing

My family makes lebkuchen at Christmastime. This tasty treat is essentially gingerbread filled with candied fruits, cut into squares, and then frosted with a drizzle of vanilla glaze. But I prefer gingerbread without the candied fruit in it. Gingerbread is seemingly the most ubiquitous holiday cookie, and I love this recipe because the cookies are soft. My children love them because they enjoy helping to cut them out. The lemon icing nicely complements the ginger and cloves in the cookies. The texture and interesting flavor combine for a great allergy-free holiday classic. MAKES ABOUT 20 COOKIES

Gingerbread Men

1²/₃ cups Chinese or superfine rice flour
¹/₂ cup potato starch
¹/₃ cup sorghum flour
1 teaspoon xanthan gum
1 teaspoon baking powder
1 tablespoon ground ginger
¹/₂ teaspoon baking soda
1¹/₂ teaspoons cinnamon
¹/₂ teaspoon cloves
¹/₂ cup organic palm fruit oil shortening
¹/₂ cup granulated sugar
¹/₄ cup applesauce
¹/₂ cup molasses
1 tablespoon cider vinegar

Lemon Icing

1 cup confectioners' sugar, sifted
1 tablespoon fresh lemon juice

1. In a large bowl whisk together the rice flour, potato starch, sorghum flour, xanthan gum, baking powder, ginger, baking soda, cinnamon, and cloves; set aside.

2. In the bowl of a stand mixer, cream the organic palm fruit oil shortening and granulated sugar until fluffy. Scrape down the sides of the bowl.

3. Add the applesauce, molasses, and cider vinegar. Beat to combine. Scrape down the sides again.

4. Slowly add the dry ingredients, mixing on low until thoroughly combined. The dough will be soft.

5. Dump the dough onto a sheet of plastic wrap and wrap it tightly. Chill the dough in the refrigerator for at least 4 hours, but preferably overnight.

6. Preheat the oven to 375°F and line two baking sheets with parchment paper.

7. Remove the chilled dough from the refrigerator and place it between two large sheets of parchment paper. Roll out the dough to a ¹/₄-inch thickness and cut with a 3-inch gingerbread man cookie cutter. Repeat this process until you have used all of the dough.

8. Place the cut cookies 1 inch apart on the prepared baking sheets and bake them in the preheated oven for 9 minutes or until they are lightly golden at the edges.

9. Remove the cookies from the oven and let them cool on the baking sheets for 10 minutes. Then remove them to cooling racks to cool completely.

10. While the cookies are cooling, make the lemon icing. Stir together the sifted confectioners' sugar and lemon juice until they are smooth and of a piping consistency. If the icing is too thick, add additional lemon juice, $1/2$ teaspoon at a time, until it is piping consistency. Load the icing into a pastry bag fitted with a #1 tip and, on completely cooled cookies, dot on the eyes, mouth, and buttons.

11. Cooled and iced cookies can be stored, refrigerated, in an airtight container for up to 5 days. They may also be frozen in an airtight container for up to 3 months.

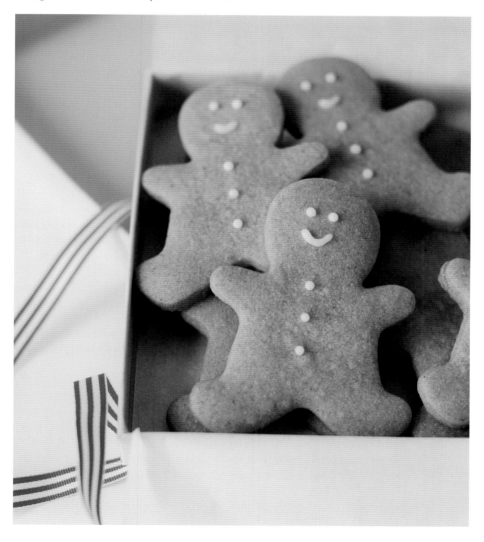

Texas Sheet Cake

My Aunt Judy makes a Texas sheet cake for my cousin Liz every year on her birthday, and, wow, do I know why. I think I only tasted my aunt's version twice before I was diagnosed with food allergies, but it was one of those desserts that I just couldn't forget. It was that good, sort of like a superrich, frosted brownie. I decided to try my hand at an allergy-free version of this beloved classic, and I am thrilled with how it turned out. This unbelievably moist and fudgy cake is so good that no one ever suspects it is allergy friendly. When I was testing this recipe, I took it to the faculty and staff at my youngest daughter's school, and they asked if I could bring more the next day! SERVES 24

Cake

1^1/$_3$ cups Chinese or superfine rice flour

^{1}/$_2$ cup potato starch

^{1}/$_4$ cup sorghum flour

1 teaspoon baking soda

2 cups sugar

^{1}/$_4$ teaspoon salt

1 teaspoon xanthan gum

1 cup organic palm fruit oil shortening

^{1}/$_3$ cup cocoa powder

1 cup water

^{1}/$_2$ cup So Delicious plain coconut milk kefir

1^1/$_2$ teaspoons vanilla extract

Frosting

^{3}/$_4$ cup organic palm fruit oil shortening

^{1}/$_2$ cup plus 1 tablespoon unsweetened cocoa powder

^{1}/$_2$ cup plus 1 tablespoon So Delicious plain, coconut milk kefir

1 pound confectioners' sugar, sifted

^{1}/$_2$ teaspoon vanilla extract

1. Preheat the oven to 350°F and lightly grease a 9 x 13-inch baking pan; set aside.

2. In a large mixing bowl, whisk together the rice flour, potato starch, sorghum flour, baking soda, sugar, salt, and xanthan gum; set aside.

3. In a large saucepan bring the organic palm fruit oil shortening, cocoa powder, and water to a boil over medium heat.

4. When the mixture boils, remove it from the heat and add it to the dry ingredients. Beat them together with a hand mixer.

5. Add the kefir and vanilla extract and stir on low until they are thoroughly incorporated. Pour the batter into the prepared pan and bake in the preheated oven for 35 minutes. When the cake comes out of the oven, let it cool in the pan on a cooling rack.

6. Meanwhile, make the frosting. Combine the palm fruit oil shortening, cocoa powder, and kefir in a saucepan and bring to a boil.

7. Remove the saucepan from the burner and beat in the sifted confectioners' sugar and vanilla extract until they are thoroughly combined.

8. Immediately pour the finished frosting over the warm cake and smooth it out with a knife. Let the cake cool completely before serving.

9. Leftovers may be stored in an airtight container, either refrigerated or at room temperature, for up to 3 days.

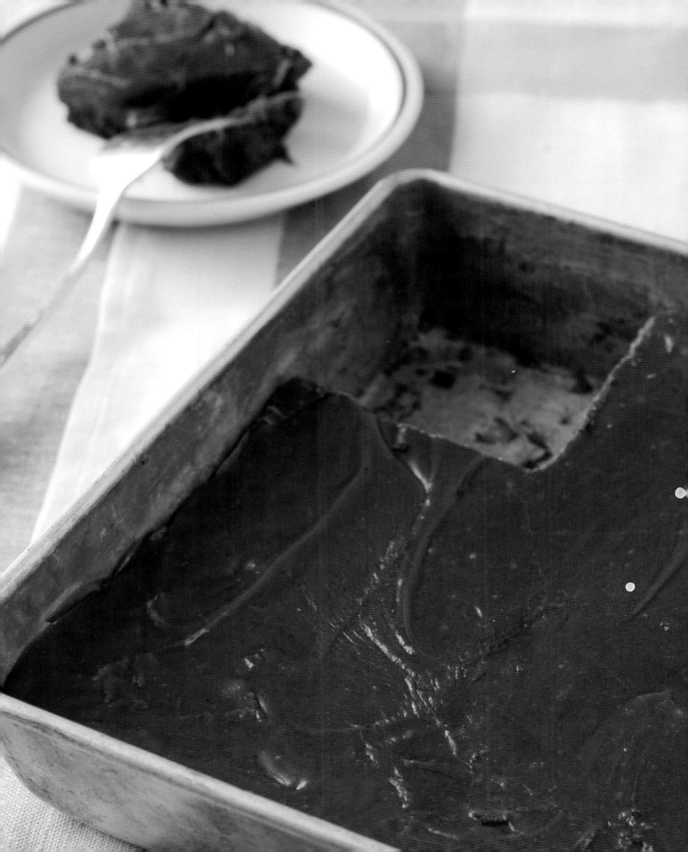

Cream-Filled Oatmeal Cookie Sandwiches

I know it's funny to make an oatmeal cookie without oatmeal, but this was one of the first flavors that I made when I started baking professionally. Back then there were no ELISA-tested oats, so oats weren't as safe for people with celiac disease. Now, with ELISA testing there are some wonderful gluten-free brands of oats, but I am still loyal to these little oat-free oatmeal cookies, not to mention the fact that they remind me of the Little Debbie Oatmeal Cream Pies™ that we used to eat when I was a little girl in Ohio. **MAKES 15 SANDWICHES**

2¼ cups Bob's Red Mill
　Gluten-Free All-Purpose
　Baking Flour*
1 teaspoon baking soda
1 teaspoon baking powder
¼ teaspoon allspice
¼ teaspoon ground cloves
½ teaspoon nutmeg
1½ teaspoons cinnamon
1 teaspoon salt
1 teaspoon xanthan gum
1 cup organic palm fruit oil
　shortening
1¼ cups dark brown sugar
¼ cup granulated sugar
2 tablespoons flaxseed meal
6 tablespoons water
1 teaspoon vanilla extract
1½ cups raisins (optional)
1 recipe Supermarket Frosting
　(see page 154)

1. Preheat the oven to 350°F. Line two baking sheets with parchment paper; set aside.

2. In a large mixing bowl, thoroughly whisk together the all-purpose baking flour, baking soda, baking powder, allspice, ground cloves, nutmeg, cinnamon, salt, and xanthan gum; set aside.

3. In the bowl of a stand mixer, cream together the organic palm fruit oil shortening and sugars.

4. While the shortening and sugars are creaming, mix together the flaxseed meal and water in a separate bowl and let stand for 1 minute. Then beat the flaxseed meal mixture and vanilla extract into the shortening and sugars and scrape down the sides of the bowl.

5. Stir in the dry ingredients and fold in the raisins.

6. Using a 1½-inch ice-cream scoop, scoop the dough onto the prepared baking sheets. Bake the cookies for 12 minutes.

7. Remove cookies from the oven and let them cool on the baking sheets for 10 minutes. Remove them to a cooling rack to cool completely before filling them with the frosting.

8. When the cookies have cooled completely, spoon about 1 tablespoon of Supermarket Frosting onto the bottom side of one of the cookies. Gently press another cookie down on top of it to form a cookie sandwich. Repeat until all the cookies are filled and sandwiched.

9. These cookies may be stored in an airtight container, refrigerated, for up to 3 to 5 days. The unfilled cookies may also be frozen in airtight containers for up to 3 months.

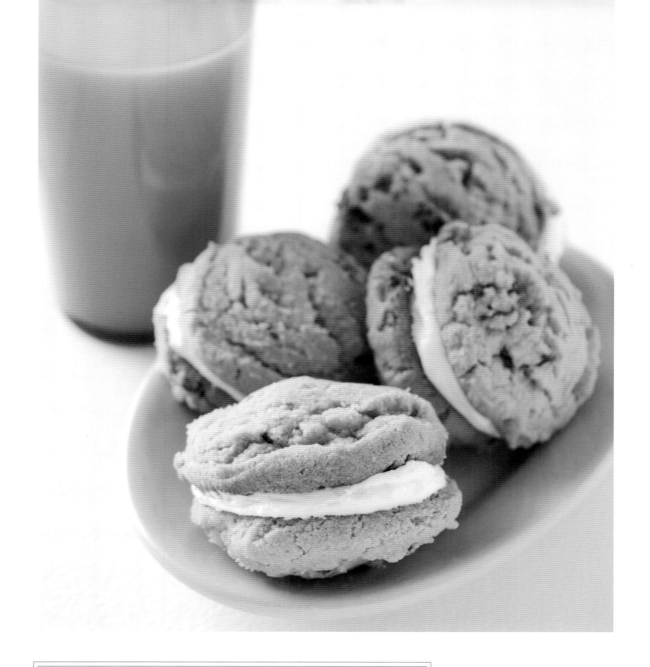

※ If you feel uncomfortable with Bob's products because of possible cross-contamination issues, please see my substitutions guide for ways to work around this product. My substitutions guide provides the weights of common gluten-free flours to make substituting easier.

Sweet Potato Pie

Last year I found myself, a week before Thanksgiving, feeling as though I couldn't eat another bite of pumpkin. Wracking my brain for a tasty alternative, I opened my cupboard and spied a can of organic sweet potato puree. Immediately, the idea of a sweet potato pie came to mind, and I realized that I had not had one since high school. Sweet and custardy, with a milder spice blend than a pumpkin pie, this was exactly the answer I was seeking to round out our Thanksgiving dinner. It was a resounding success, and I think that your family will enjoy it just as much as ours did. SERVES 10–12

1 Basic Double Piecrust (see page 161)
2 cups pureed sweet potato
1/2 cup light brown sugar
1/2 cup granulated sugar
1 1/2 teaspoons cinnamon
1/4 teaspoon nutmeg
1/2 teaspoon salt
1 cup So Delicious plain coconut milk creamer
1/4 cup plus 2 teaspoons cornstarch

1. Preheat the oven to 350°F.

2. Make the Basic Double Piecrust according to the recipe directions, reserving half for another use. Press the remaining half of the crust into a 9-inch pie plate, crimp the edges, and prick it all over with a fork. Place a greased piece of tin foil directly over the top of the crust and weight the foil with dried beans or pie weights. Bake the crust, covered with the foil, in the preheated oven for 8 minutes. Remove the foil from the crust and return it to the oven for about 5 more minutes or until the bottom of the crust appears just dry.

3. While the piecrust is baking, mix together the sweet potato puree, light brown sugar, granulated sugar, cinnamon, nutmeg, and salt.

4. In a separate, small bowl, whisk together the creamer and cornstarch until smooth. Add the creamer mixture to the sweet potato filling. Whisk until it is smooth and all of the ingredients are thoroughly combined.

5. Pour the sweet potato filling into the prepared piecrust. Return the pie to the oven to bake for 60 minutes or until the custard is set. If the crust begins to brown too quickly, cover the edges with foil.

6. Completely cool the pie on a cooling rack before cutting. Store leftovers, covered and refrigerated, for up to 3 days. You can make the pie up to 2 days in advance; cover and store it in the refrigerator until ready to serve.

Note: If this pie isn't completely cool before cutting, the filling will ooze. I let mine cool overnight before attacking it.

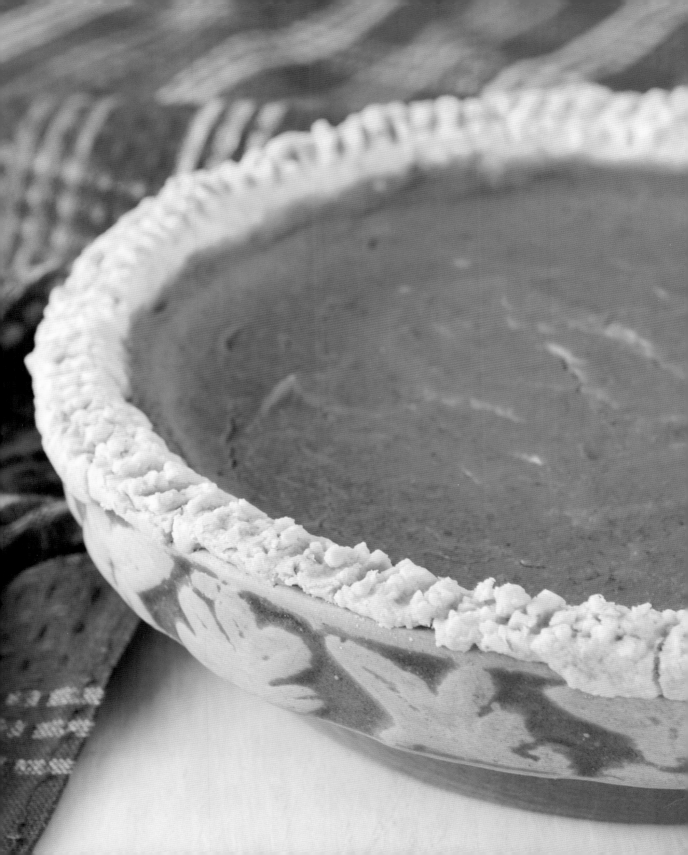

Not Really Peanut Butter Fudge

Creamy, rich, and perfect for packing up for friends and family for the holidays, this delicious fudge is so good you will never suspect there is no peanut butter in it. When I made these, I noticed they mysteriously vanished from the refrigerator very quickly. My sneaky family just kept going back for more—they were so surprised that it wasn't made with peanut butter. For those with peanut allergies, the sunflower seed butter serves as a supertasty substitute, but if you cannot tolerate sunflower seed butter, you may use your preferred peanut butter alternative instead. Because this fudge is made with coconut oil, make sure to keep it refrigerated. Coconut oil has a very low melting point, and the fudge will otherwise soften. MAKES 36 PIECES

½ **cup coconut oil (measured in its solid form)**
2 cups brown sugar
½ **cup So Delicious plain coconut milk creamer**
⅔ **cup sunflower seed butter**
1 teaspoon vanilla extract
3 cups confectioners' sugar, sifted

1. Lightly grease an 8 x 8-inch square pan; set aside.

2. In a medium saucepan melt the coconut oil over low heat. Stir in the brown sugar and creamer and turn the heat up to medium-high. Stirring constantly, bring the mixture to a boil and let it boil for 2 minutes.

3. Remove the mixture from the heat and stir in the sunflower seed butter and vanilla extract.

4. Stir in the confectioners' sugar until the fudge is smooth.

5. Pour the fudge into the prepared pan and refrigerate it for 4 hours or until it is solid. When ready, cut the fudge with a hot knife.

6. Store the fudge in an airtight container, refrigerated, for up to 7 days.

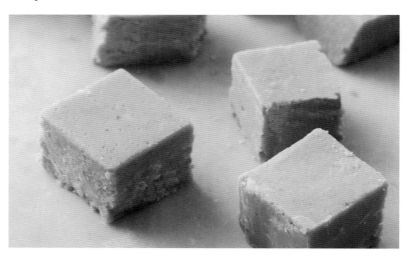

Chocolate Egg Cream

Before I moved to New York City, I had no idea what an egg cream was. Like most people, I think, I assumed it was something made with meringue, or at least something actually made with eggs. I might never have tried one were it not for the fact that when my husband and I were first dating, he drank one every time we went to a diner. I was sort of disgusted by the idea of milk mixed with seltzer, but once I tried it, I was sold. This tasty dairy-free version is just as delicious as the real thing. Make sure you use fresh seltzer and not club soda to make it. SERVES 1

1. Pour the chocolate syrup into a tall glass. Add the vanilla rice milk and stir vigorously until the chocolate is completely stirred in.

2. Pour in the seltzer and quickly stir to combine. Drink the egg cream immediately.

¼ **cup chocolate syrup (see Where to Shop)**
⅓ **cup vanilla rice milk**
1 cup fresh seltzer

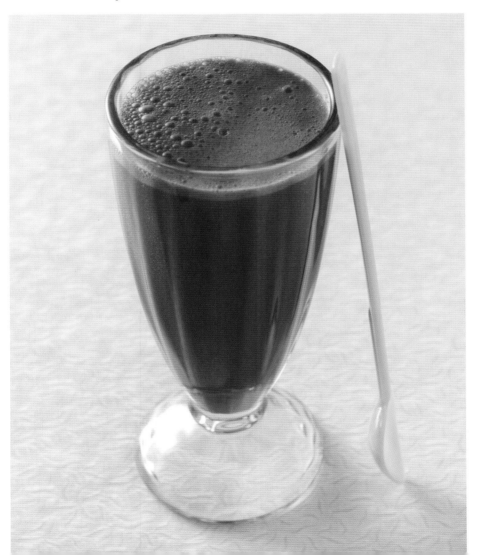

Snickerdoodles

My grandmother on my dad's side rarely baked, but when she did, she made snickerdoodles. I love them. I know that many people prefer chocolate to cinnamon, but I'll take something sweet and cinnamony over something chocolaty any day of the week. These cookies are just right in their texture and level of cinnamon sweetness. These are sure to be an after-school or lunchbox favorite. **MAKES 30 COOKIES**

$^{1}/_{3}$ cup granulated sugar

$^{3}/_{4}$ teaspoon cinnamon

2$^{1}/_{4}$ cups Bob's Red Mill Gluten-Free All-Purpose Baking Flour*

1 teaspoon baking soda

1 teaspoon baking powder

1 teaspoon xanthan gum

1 teaspoon salt

1 cup organic palm fruit oil shortening

$^{3}/_{4}$ cup brown sugar

$^{3}/_{4}$ cup granulated sugar

2 tablespoons ground flaxseed meal

2 tablespoons water

1 teaspoon vanilla extract

1. Preheat the oven to 350°F. Line two baking sheets with parchment paper; set aside.

2. In a small bowl mix together the $^{1}/_{3}$ cup sugar and cinnamon; set aside.

3. In a large bowl, whisk together the all-purpose baking flour, baking soda, baking powder, xanthan gum, and salt.

4. In the bowl of a stand mixer, cream together the organic palm fruit oil shortening and the sugars until light and fluffy.

5. While the shortening and sugars are creaming, mix together the flaxseed meal and the water in a small bowl. Stop the mixer and scrape down the bowl. Add the flaxseed meal mixture and vanilla extract. Beat the batter again. Scrape down the sides again and then slowly stir in the dry ingredients.

6. Using a 1$^{1}/_{2}$-inch ice-cream scoop, scoop the dough and then roll it between your hands to form a ball. Roll each dough ball in the sugar and cinnamon mixture until thoroughly coated.

7. Place the coated balls 2 inches apart on the prepared baking sheets. Bake the cookies in the preheated oven for 12 minutes.

8. Remove the trays from the oven and let the cookies cool for 10 minutes on the baking sheets and then remove them to cooling racks to cool completely.

9. These cookies may be stored in airtight containers, at room temperature, for up to 3 days, or they may be frozen in airtight containers for up to 3 months.

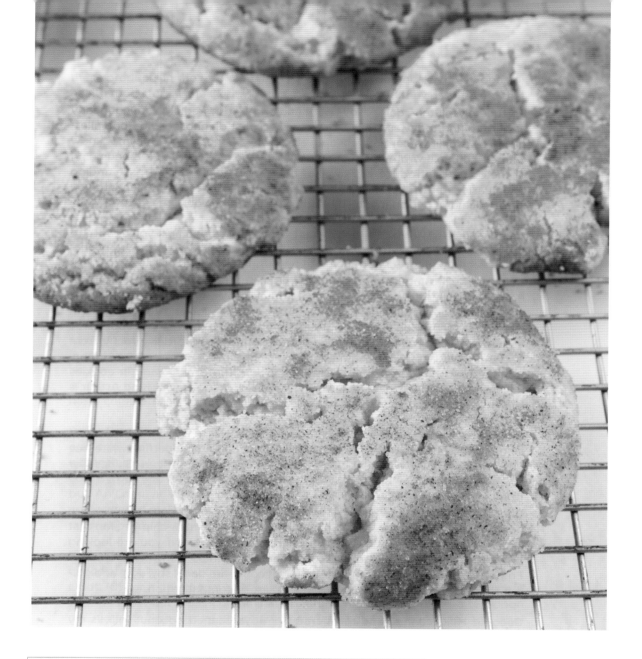

✳ If you feel uncomfortable with Bob's products because of possible cross-contamination issues, please see my substitutions guide for ways to work around this product. My substitutions guide provides the weights of common gluten-free flours to make substituting easier.

French Lentils—In some areas, you can find French lentils at regular supermarkets. In others they are only available at specialty stores like Zabar's and Dean & Deluca and online at places like Amazon and Bob's Red Mill.

Gluten-Free Cornflakes—I especially like the Nature's Path Organic, Fruit Juice–Sweetened Corn Flakes, which are gluten-free. They are available at Whole Foods Markets, health food stores, and supermarkets nationwide. If you cannot find them in your local store, please check Amazon or ask your supermarket manager to special order them. If this seems like too much work, substitute Rice or Corn Chex for the cornflakes.

Gluten-Free Hamburger Buns—There are a couple of brands of gluten-free hamburger buns available. However, the trick for me is to find a brand that is also egg free. Whole Foods Gluten-Free Bakehouse, available at Whole Foods Markets nationwide, or Ener-G White Rice Hamburger Buns are two such brands. Ener-G White Rice Hamburger Buns are available at health food stores and supermarkets nationwide or on Amazon.

Gluten- and Soy-Free Deli Meats, Bacon, and Hot Dogs—My favorite brand is Applegate Farms because it is easy to find in New York City. I also love Wellshire Farms. Both may be found at Whole Foods Markets nationwide and in many local supermarkets as well.

Leaf Lard—Good, nonhydrogenated leaf lard is hard to find these days, but it really makes a difference. Lard that you find at the supermarket does not have the same flavor as fresh, nonhydrogenated leaf lard, but instead it has a stronger pork flavor. I do not recommend it. Instead, try looking at your local farmers' market or at Prairie Pride Farm of Minnesota (www.prairiepridepork .com/leaflard.php).

Lyle's Golden Syrup—In both New York and California, Lyle's is available at most major supermarkets, so I am assuming that it is also available, for the most part, nationwide. It is definitely available in Europe. If you cannot find it in your area, it is available on Amazon.

Maldon Salt—Maldon is available in most supermarkets, specialty stores, and natural food stores nationwide.

Masa Harina—Masa harina is a finely ground white corn flour used in many Latin American dishes. Bob's Red Mill makes a version that is readily available at supermarkets nationwide as well as on Amazon. If you cannot find the Bob's version, another popular and authentic brand is Maseca. If you cannot find Maseca at your local supermarket, you can get it online at Amazon.

Mustard—Having lived in France for a little while, I became spoiled when it came to mustard. In the United States, I love Maille mustard, and this is the brand that I am referring to throughout the book when I say "good" mustard. Maille is available in most local supermarkets. If you cannot find it, ask your supermarket manager if he or she would consider stocking it, or buy it online on Amazon.

Oil Mister—Several times throughout the book, I refer to misting or spraying a recipe with a little oil. I recommend the Misto Stainless Steel Oil Sprayer. You can find it at the Container Store or online at Amazon. This ensures that what you are using is 100 percent canola or olive oil without a soy-based propellant.

Organic Palm Fruit Oil Shortening—Organic palm fruit oil shortening is easy to find in New York City, but it isn't always as easy to find everywhere else. In New York, I find it at Whole Foods Markets and at our local health food stores. In Ohio, I find it at Kroger. In California, I found it at Whole Foods Market and Jungle Jim's International Market. Both Whole Foods and Jungle Jim's make their own brands of palm fruit oil shortening, too. If you cannot find this kind of shortening in your area, try buying Spectrum Organic Shortening online from Amazon. You can also get organic palm shortening from a website called Tropical Traditions (www.tropicaltraditions.com/organic_palm_shortening.htm). And, before you give up entirely, make sure that you flip over your package of "all vegetable shortening." Sometimes vegetable shortening is not clearly marked as organic palm fruit oil on the front of the package.

Quinoa Flakes—Ancient Harvest quinoa flakes and regular Aztec red quinoa are my favorite quinoa products. You can get Ancient Harvest products at most supermarkets nationwide, at health food stores, or on Amazon. I have even seen this brand at my corner deli!

Sorghum Beer—I used Red Bridge Gluten-Free Sorghum Beer when I tested the recipes in this book, but you may use any gluten-free beer you prefer. I found it at Whole Foods Market, but it is also available online on Amazon.

Sorghum Flour—In the United States, sorghum flour is available just about anywhere that Bob's Red Mill products are sold. If you are having trouble finding it, you can also order it online at www.authenticfoods.com.

Sprinkles and Sanding Sugars—I recommend using India Tree products because they use natural vegetable dyes and do not process nuts in their facility. Look for everything from multicolored sanding sugar to egg-free candied violets to food coloring on their website, www.indiatree.com. The website also offers a detailed list of ingredients and possible allergens for every product they sell. I also like "Let's Do . . . Sprinkelz" brand confetti sprinkles.

Sunflower Seed Butter—I prefer the SunButter sunflower seed butter because it is made in a dedicated nut-free facility. It is available at Whole Foods Market and online at Amazon. It is, however, run on a line that also processes soy. Though the line is thoroughly cleaned, if you are severely soy-allergic, you can also grind your own sunflower butter in a food processor.

Xanthan Gum—It has recently come to my attention that one of my favorite brands of xanthan gum is now being grown on soy. This is a great example of why it's important to always check the ingredients label when shopping; companies can and do change their ingredients without warning. Ener-G brand makes a soy-free version that you can order online through Amazon or directly through their website, http://www.ener-g.com/.

Xylitol—You can find this sweetener at Whole Foods Market, health food stores, Amazon, and the Vitamin Shop. Make sure to keep it well out of reach of pets and do not let them eat any finished products made with xylitol. While xylitol is completely natural and safe for human consumption, it is deadly to dogs and cats.

Acknowledgments

I wish I could claim total credit for this book, but the truth is that without the help of so many people, I never could have made it a reality. Thank you, first, to my husband, Jesse, who not only tasted and critiqued every recipe, but who also tolerated the late nights and distracted the kids so that I could finish my work. I am also grateful to my girls, Margot and Colombe, who, again, sacrificed much time with me so that I could get this done. Carmen gets a big thank you for her assistance with everything. Marni Salup deserves a huge round of applause for her continued support and everything else she does behind the scenes. Thank you to Dorthea Casselman for never making me feel like a dunce when I asked her the same math questions over and over again. She cheerfully responded, and these recipes could not have happened without her assistance with ratios. Maija and Steve, well, I owe you for never saying that you were full and for being so diligent about returning the Tupperware. Thank you Tamar Rydzinski for fielding my questions, listening to my ideas, and believing in my work. You always make me feel supported even when you have to disagree with me. Lara Asher, thank you doesn't seem adequate. You will never know how much I appreciate your warmth and enthusiasm. It has truly been a pleasure.

Index

About the Author

Elizabeth Gordon is the author of *Allergy-Free Desserts: Gluten-Free, Dairy-Free, Egg-Free, Soy-Free, and Nut-Free Delights* and a full-time mother. Inspired to write cookbooks by her own food allergies, she lives in New York City with her husband and children. For more information and additional recipes, go to Elizabeth's website, www.myallergyfreelifestyle, or her blog, www.allergyfreedelights.com.